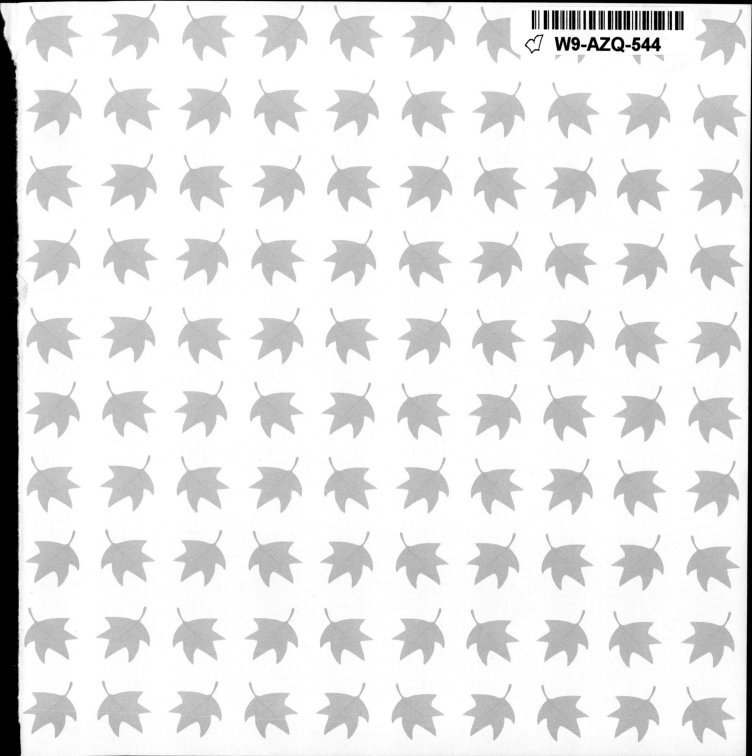

THE MASSAGE MANUAL

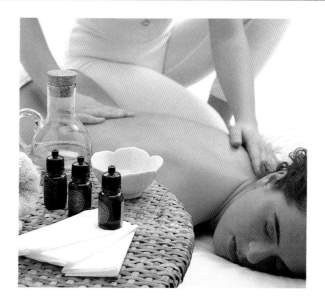

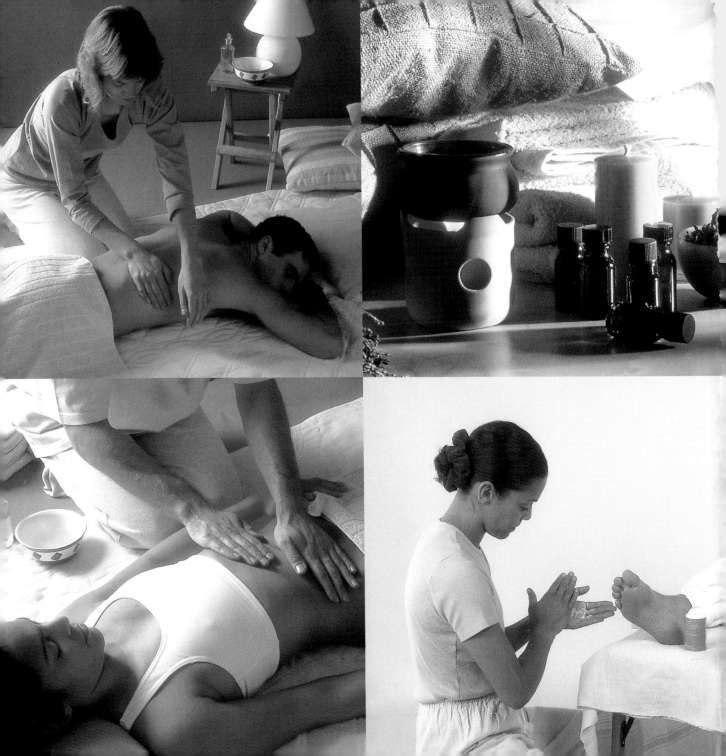

THE MASSAGE MANUAL

Massage • Aromatherapy • Shiatsu • Reflexology

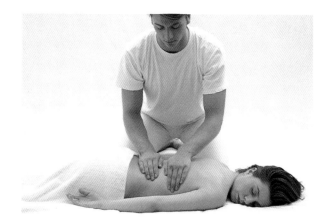

MARK EVANS, SUZANNE FRANZEN, ROSALIND OXENFORD

HERMES
HOUSE

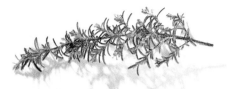

First published in 1999 by Hermes House

© Anness Publishing Limited 1999

Hermes House is an imprint of Anness Publishing Limited
Hermes House, 88-89 Blackfriars Road
London SE1 8HA

This edition published in the USA by Hermes House,
Anness Publishing Inc., 27 West 20th Street, New York, NY10011;
(800) 354-9657

ISBN 1 84038 227 9

A CIP catalogue record for this book is available from the British Library

Publisher: Joanna Lorenz
Project Editor: Fiona Eaton
Editor: Emma Gray
Additional text: Nitya Lacroix and Sharon Seager
Jacket Designer: Simon Wilder
Designers: Bobbie Colgate Stone and Allan Mole
Illustrator: Michael Shoebridge
Photographer: Don Last
Editorial Reader: Felicity Forster
Production Controller: Don Campaniello

Previously published as four separate volumes, *Instant Massage, Instant Aromatherapy, Reflexology* and *Shiatsu*

Printed and bound in Singapore

1 3 5 7 9 10 8 6 4 2

The reader should not regard the recommendations, ideas and techniques expressed and described in this book as substitutes
for the advice of a qualified medical practitioner or other qualified professional. Any use to which the recommendations, ideas and
techniques are put is at the reader's sole discretion and risk.

CONTENTS

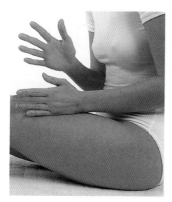

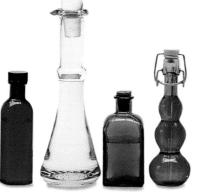

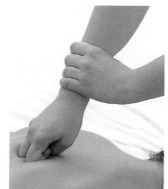

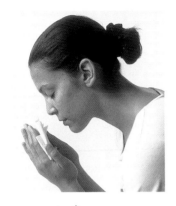

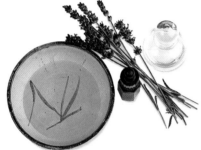

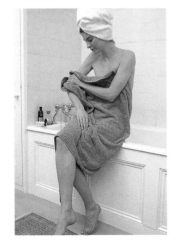

THE POWER OF SCENT: THE ART OF AROMATHERAPY 78

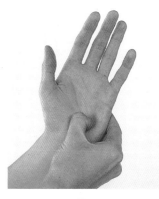

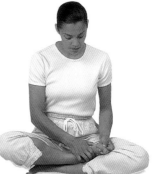

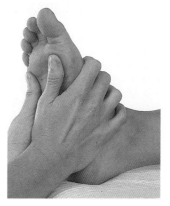

INTRODUCTION

DO YOU COME HOME at the end of the day with your neck and shoulders feeling as if they were set in concrete? Does stress leave your back stiff and aching? If you get angry and tense, do you clench your fists, leaving your hands and arms heavy and tired? Anyone who has experienced the physical tensions that can accompany stressful situations will probably not be surprised to learn that massage is one of the most successful ways to relax painful, knotted muscles.

THE POWER OF TOUCH

Most of us almost unconsciously rub tense, aching muscles to get

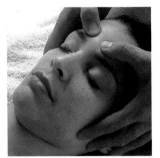

some instant relief; correctly performed, massage can have a wonderful effect, not just on the muscles themselves but on our whole sense of well-being. Touch is one of the most crucial, and yet often neglected, senses and the need for human touch remains constant throughout life. In the last thirty years, many studies have looked at the importance of touch for human development. In one of these, premature babies who were gently stroked for 45 minutes a day were found to be nearly 50 per cent heavier after ten days than those who were not; they were also more active, alert and responsive.

Systematic, caring touch through massage movements has been shown to encourage the release of endorphins – chemicals that affect development in children and emotional and physical well-being in adults. Studies show that people who experience frequent touch live longer and have fewer ailments. Professional massage can be an effective treatment for a range of physical problems and is a wonderfully relaxing experience. Many simple techniques can also be used at home to help ease both your own and other people's tensions. By following the suggestions in this book, you can reassure, relax and comfort your family or friends in a way that no non-touch therapy can do. When you consider that an area of skin the size of a coin contains over three million cells, 50 nerve endings and some 90 cm (3 ft) of blood vessels, you can see how much impact touch can have on people.

the nervous system. In reflexology, as in acupuncture, places or points relate to or reflect organs of the body.

Treatment of the feet and hands and of pressure points has been practised for thousands of years, the earliest known evidence being an Egyptian relief dated around 2,500–2,300 BC. The feet were worked in ancient China in conjunction with acupuncture, being treated first to stimulate the whole body and find areas of disturbance, and acupuncture needles then being applied as fine tuning. Foot treatment was also practised in India and Indonesia and among Native Americans, who hold a central belief that our feet are our connection with the earth and the earth's energies.

In Europe, pressure point therapy was used from the Middle Ages, but it was not until this century that Westerners explored and developed knowledge of reflexology and brought together the wisdom and practices of the ancient cultures with our modern understanding of the subject.

ESSENTIAL OILS IN MASSAGE THERAPY

When the therapeutic touch of massage is used in conjunction with potent essential oils, the treatment works on both mind and body, mainly on the nervous system, and is able both to relax and stimulate. The oils penetrate the body via the

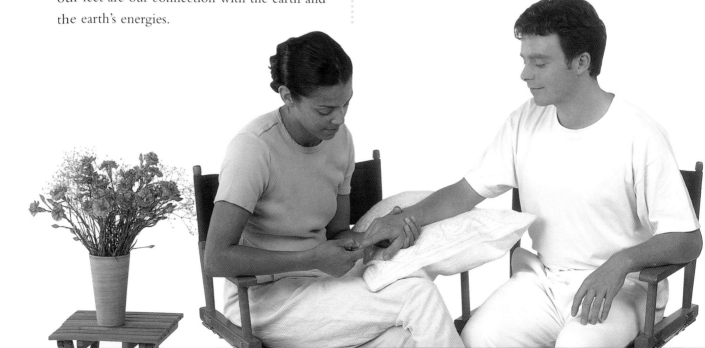

skin and are also inhaled during treatment. The sense of smell has the most subtle significance in our lives. Most of the pleasure we derive from foods stems from their aroma; the initial attraction of other people probably depends on their scent as much as anything else.

Moods can be enhanced or changed with the use of scents. Aromatic plants contain essential oils that have been used for centuries to relax, sedate, refresh or stimulate according to need. Airborne aromatic molecules are detected by the brain's olfactory centre via the nostrils, and produce an immediate emotional or instinctive response from the limbic system within the brain.

Aromatic essential oils can have significant physiological and pharmacological effects as well as affecting mood. Aromatic molecules may enter the lungs and become absorbed into the bloodstream which can carry them to all parts of the body, or they may be absorbed into the bloodstream when used with massage oils via the skin. Each aromatic oil has its own individual combination of constituents and these in turn can interact with the body's chemistry to have specific therapeutic effects.

THE DEVELOPMENT OF AROMATHERAPY

The origins and development of our knowledge of aromatic oils coincide with the history of mankind. Ancient written records, whether they be the Vedic manuscripts from India dating back some 3,000 years, Egyptian papyri from 1,500 BC or biblical stories of the Jewish exodus from Egypt about 300 years later, all describe the widespread use of aromatic oils for religious ceremonies and rituals as well as in massage, baths and for scenting the hair and body.

The invention of the distillation process is generally credited to Arabic physicians of the tenth century AD, though it may have been known much earlier. Certainly, the Arabic use of concentrated, distilled oils led to a renaissance in the use of aromatic plants. In the West, there was a gradual separation of perfumery and more medical applications; the latter led to synthetic chemistry, and a loss of the sense of the psychological aspects of aroma.

When the French chemist, René-Maurice Gattefosse, burnt his hand and accidentally discovered the healing powers of lavender oil, he began to investigate essential oils and discovered that they were often more effective than isolated or synthetic compounds. In 1928 he coined the term "aromatherapy" to describe the use of aromatic oils for treating physical or emotional problems. During World War II, essential oils were used to treat conditions ranging from infections and diseases to psychiatric disorders. This kind of work started to bridge the gap that had grown between the physical properties and emotional effects of therapy.

Aromatherapists today may use specific essential oils for their physiological effects, but there is no reason why these may not also be used for their relaxing properties, if used carefully. Essential oils are often produced by plants as part of their defences against predators, and they should always be treated with respect. In this book the focus is on their role in stress reduction.

THE BENEFITS OF MASSAGE

Giving a massage or other physical therapy to another person is a privilege, as you are being allowed to make direct contact with their inner being. Just placing your hands on someone else's body can give them a strong sense of relaxation and can release blocked energy. It is also an opportunity to connect with the energy of another person and can increase your own sensitivity. Shared touch with your partner helps to make your relationship grow and deepen. All in all, one of the best routes for deeper relaxation, more vitality and greater self-awareness is through massage.

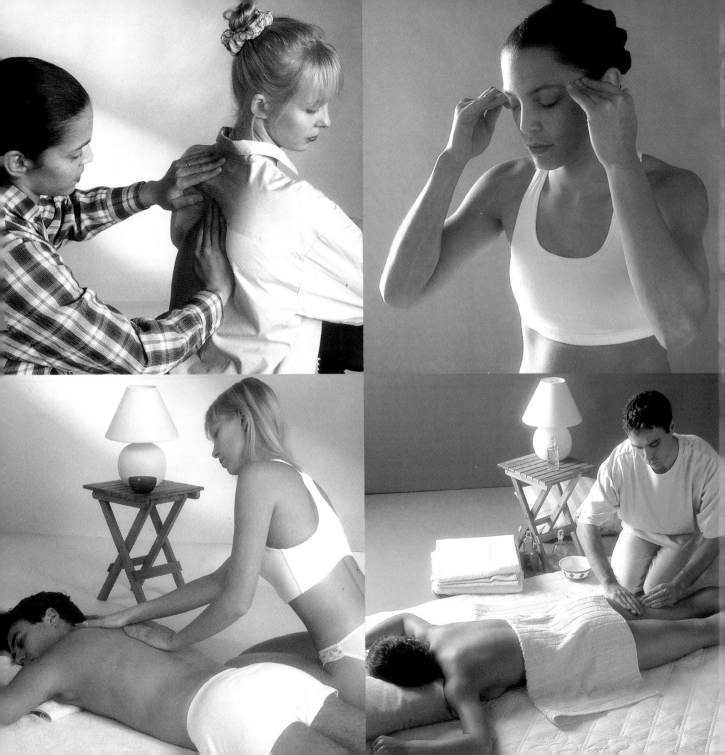

THE HEALING TOUCH: *the Art of Massage*

THE SENSE OF TOUCH is a powerful and highly sensitive form of communication. It is a natural reaction to reach out and touch, whether to feel an object or to respond to – perhaps to comfort – another person. When applied with skill and care, massage can evoke many beneficial changes within the body, mind and spirit. As the strokes ease pain and tension from aching muscles, boost a sluggish circulation and eliminate accumulated toxic matter, the nurturing touch of the hands soothes away mental stress and restores emotional equilibrium.

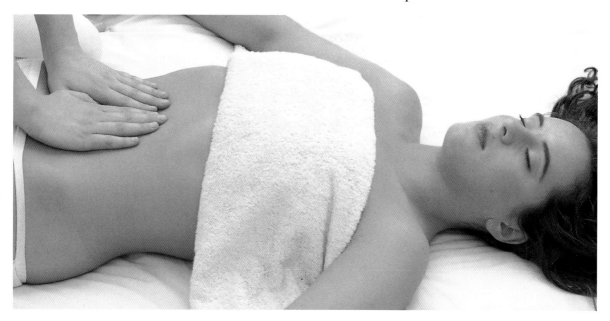

PREPARING FOR MASSAGE

CREATING THE RIGHT ENVIRONMENT and space for treatment can contribute to making massage an even more relaxing and beneficial experience. Before you start, make sure that the room is pleasantly warm and the area for massage is padded enough for your partner to be truly comfortable. Have some towels or a sheet handy to cover areas not being worked on – remember that if you are working on the floor, draughts can give exposed flesh very unrelaxing goose-pimples. If you are using oil, place it in a convenient spot where you can reach it easily without the risk of knocking it over.

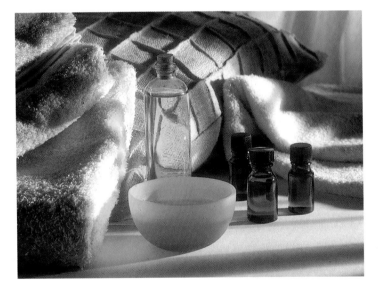

Preparing yourself is important too; physically this means removing watches and jewellery from your hands and wrists and wearing loose, comfortable clothing, ideally short-sleeved. Try to do a few stretches and take a few deep breaths to help you to feel calm; if you give a massage when you are tense yourself, this may be transmitted to your massage partner. This can work the other way round too, so feel prepared mentally to let go of any tensions that you feel coming from the other person's body and avoid absorbing his or her stresses.

When using oil, pour it on to your own hands first to warm it up, never directly on to your partner. The oil may be placed in a bowl, glass bottle or squeezy bottle for ease of use. Spread oil slowly on to the body – and then begin.

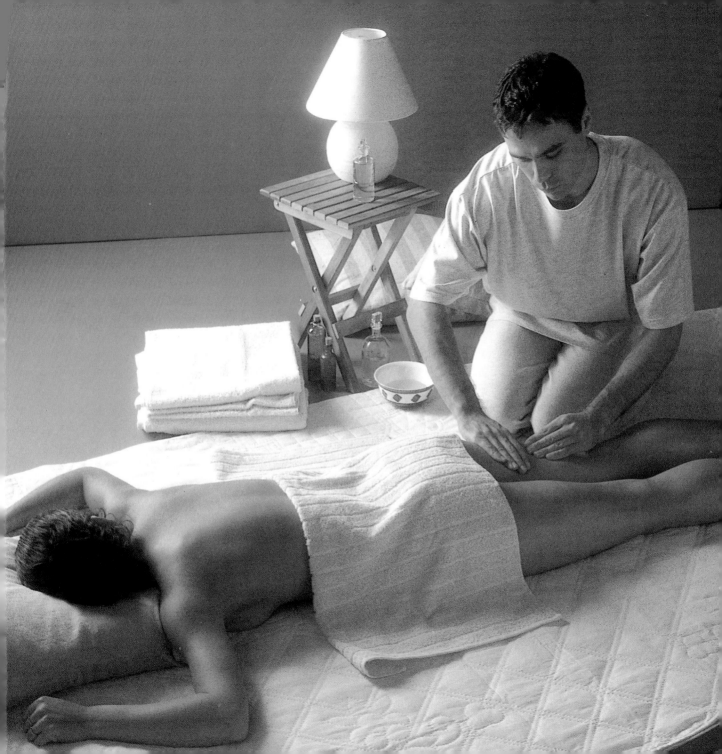

MASSAGE OILS

Massage is a wonderful way to use essential oils, suitably diluted in a good base oil, for your partner or family. Use soft, thick towels to cover areas of the body you are not massaging, and make sure that the room is warm, perhaps with an additional portable heater.

Suitable base oils include sweet almond oil (probably the most versatile and useful), grapeseed, safflower, soya (a bit thicker and stickier), coconut and even sunflower. For very dry skins, a small amount of jojoba, avocado or wheatgerm oils (except in cases of wheat allergy) may be added. Essential oils may be blended at a dilution of 1 per cent, or one drop per 5 ml (1 tsp) of base oil; this may sometimes be increased to 2 per cent, but take care that no skin reactions occur with any oil.

CAUTION:
If someone has sensitive skin or suffers from allergies, then try massaging with just one drop of essential oil per 20 ml (4 tsp) of base oil at first to test for any reaction (rare). Seek medical advice before massaging a pregnant woman.

Right: One of the nicest ways of using aromatic essential oils is diluted in a base massage oil.

MIXING ESSENTIAL OILS FOR MASSAGE

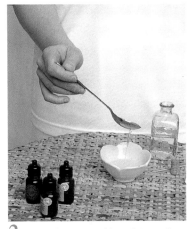

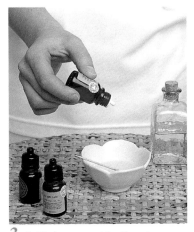

1 Before you begin, wash and dry your hands and make sure that all the utensils are clean and dry. Measure out about 10 ml (2 tsp) of your chosen vegetable oil.

2 Pour the vegetable oil into the blending bowl.

3 Add the essential oil, a drop at a time. Mix with a cocktail stick.

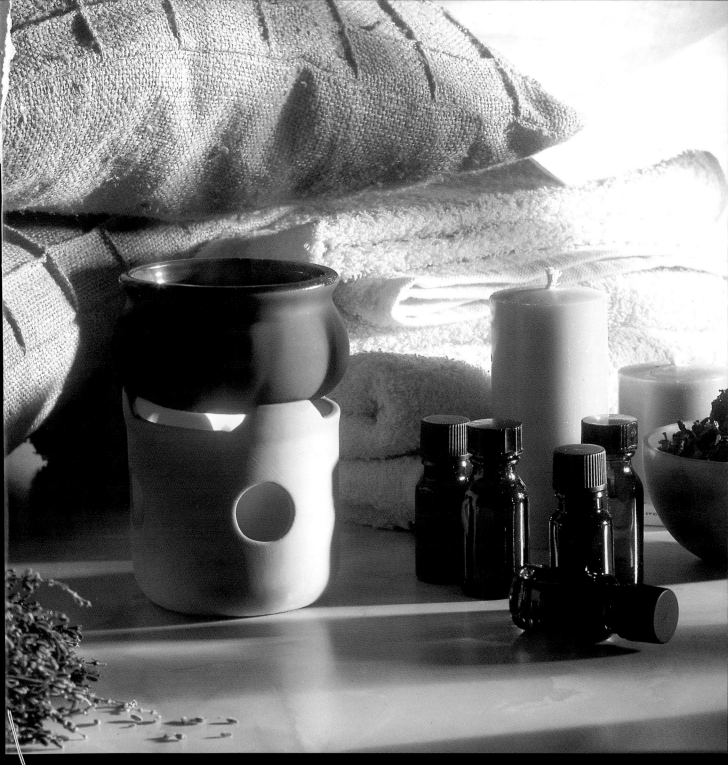

BASIC STROKES

There are many different kinds of massage movements that have specific effects on the body; the basic strokes that form the main substance of massage can, however, be included in a few categories or types. The pattern of a massage often follows certain fundamental principles. To begin with there is the initial contact; the calm, unhurried and relaxed way that you first touch your massage partner can in itself lay the foundation for a soothing, unwinding experience.

GLIDING

A massage usually starts with slow, broad and relatively superficial movements, leading to deeper and perhaps more specific techniques on smaller areas of spasm or tension. If the person needs invigorating or toning up, then faster movements may be used, and finally more soothing, stretching or stroking movements can help to finish the massage in a relaxed way.

The first and last of the massage movements are often therefore gliding strokes. In professional massage parlance these are called effleurage, and involve long, soothing moves that cover a wide area – for instance, the whole of the back. It is perfectly possible to give a complete massage with these stroking techniques, and for gentle relaxation this may be best.

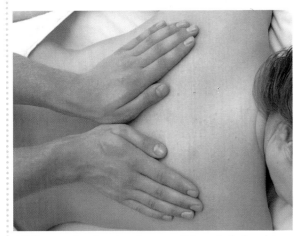

Gliding strokes involve the use of the whole hand in smooth movements.

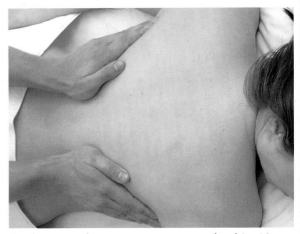

Apply even pressure as you move over the skin. Use plenty of oil.

CIRCLING

An allied form of movement is circling, where the hands move large areas of muscle in a circular motion. Since tension within muscles can produce knotted areas that may need working along or across the length of the fibres, this circular action starts to release the knots before deeper movements are used.

Circling may be carried out with just one hand, or both hands can be used, one on top of the other, for greater depth and stability of action. Like the gliding motions, circling is essentially a slow, relaxing type of movement and should not be rushed.

As with all massage strokes, try to keep your own body comfortable and unstrained, and avoid tensing your hands or arms. Keep a good balance, with your legs slightly apart to enable you to move rhythmically.

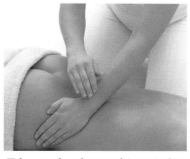

A variation on simple circling uses both hands.

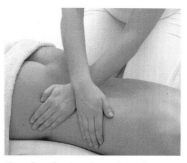

Take one hand around in a circle, then the other.

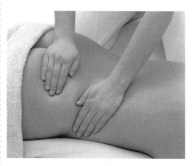

Overlap the hands so that they follow one another smoothly.

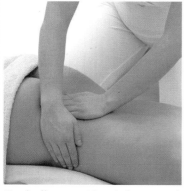

Gradually move the circles up and down the back.

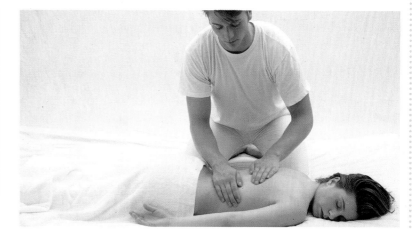

KNEADING

After the recipient has been relaxed by steady stroking or gliding movements and tense muscles start to release, a professional massage therapist may well begin to use deeper techniques to soften the knotted areas. The general term for many of these movements is petrissage, and they involve a squeezing action to encourage waste matter to be pumped out of the muscles and allow fresh, oxygenated blood to flow in.

The most well-known and widely used of these techniques is kneading. This has some similarities to kneading dough, with the thumbs working on small areas to squeeze the flesh and ease out the tense knots. The movement can be a little tricky to apply correctly at first, but when mastered it is a really useful way to revitalize tired, stiff muscles quickly.

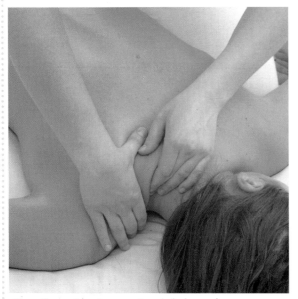

Kneading with alternate hands helps to loosen tense, knotted muscles.

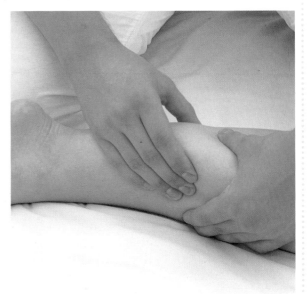

On smaller areas like the calves, use less pressure to avoid discomfort.

WRINGING

Another important petrissage-type of movement is wringing, where the action of one hand against the other creates a powerful squeezing action. When performed on the back for example, the person's own spine acts as a block against which the muscles are wrung. This enables the speedy removal of waste matter from tense muscles.

All muscular activity produces potentially toxic waste materials, notably lactic acid. If the person also gets tense and stiff, these wastes are trapped within the muscles, making them even stiffer and aching more. Wringing is a very effective way of encouraging the drainage of lactic acid and other waste matter, which in turn allows new blood to flood in, bringing oxygen and fresh nutrients to each cell.

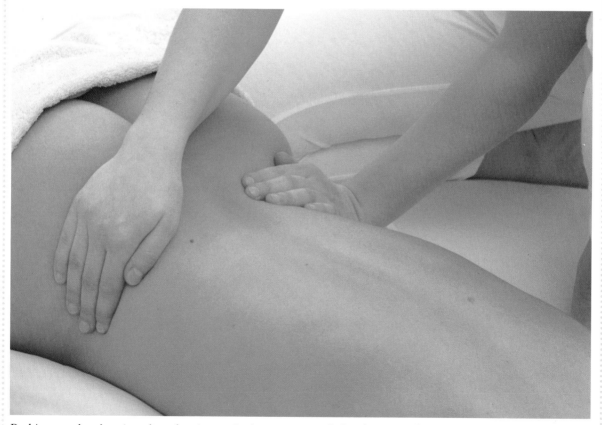

Pushing one hand against the other in a wringing movement helps the removal of waste matter.

PRESSURE TECHNIQUES

As a massage treatment progresses, general techniques such as gliding and circling often change into more detailed and specific work on smaller areas of real spasm. Professional massage therapists may move from petrissage movements to even deeper work with firm pressure using the thumbs or fingers.

In general, pressure techniques are less painful when performed along the direction of the muscle fibres, rather than across them. Pressure is achieved by steadily leaning into the movement with the whole body, not by tensing your hands. The depth of the pressure applied should be adjusted for individual comfort; usually thinner people need lighter pressure.

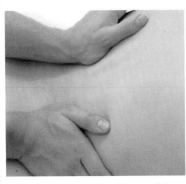

Deeper pressures may be used in professional massage.

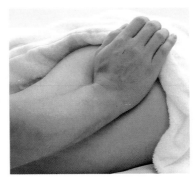

The heel of the hand gives a broad, firm effect.

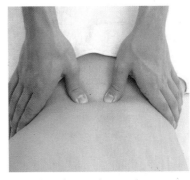

The thumbs can be used to exert the most precise pressure.

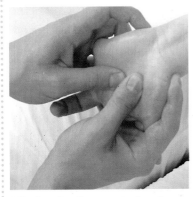

The hands often respond well to firm work.

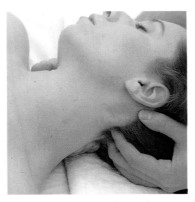

Careful pressure to the neck muscles can give much relief.

CAUTION:

Do not attempt deep work if at all unsure of the effect, or if pain occurs. Underdo rather than overdo massage – effleurage and petrissage movements can make a complete and thoroughly relaxing massage.

PERCUSSION

If someone has a generally sluggish system, or needs invigorating, say before exercise, then faster techniques may be useful. The overall term for these strokes is percussion, or tapotement. Unlike any of the other strokes described here, they need to be performed quickly, to stimulate circulation under the skin and tone the associated muscles.

One of the best known of these movements is hacking, where the sides of the fingers are used to flick rhythmically up and down to create a slightly stinging sensation. Despite being shown frequently in filmed scenes of massage, this and other percussive movements are not at all a major part of massage, but they do have a number of useful effects.

Cupping is another similar stroke which helps to bring blood to the area being worked on. This technique is often used in treating medical conditions such as cystic fibrosis, where a lot of thick, sticky mucus can build up in the lungs. Cupping on the back can help to loosen this mucus enabling it to be brought up and out of the body by the cough reflex.

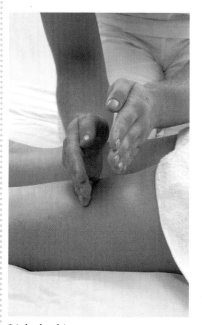

Light hacking movements stimulate the circulation.

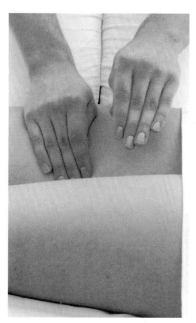

Cupping is another good percussion technique.

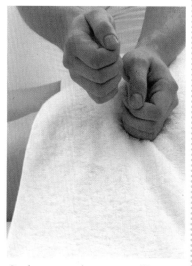

On large muscles, pummelling with loose fists will help to tone and invigorate.

SELF-MASSAGE

ONE OF THE NICEST THINGS about massage is that you do not need to invest in expensive equipment to do many of the movements, and indeed several strokes can also be successfully used for self-massage. The advantage of working on your own muscles is that you will know exactly how deeply you can press, getting instant feedback from your body about the effects of the massage. Obviously it is not possible to do a complete self-massage, and therapeutically it cannot equal the experience of relaxing on a couch and surrendering yourself to a professional massage treatment. However, you will find that there are many times when you can help yourself

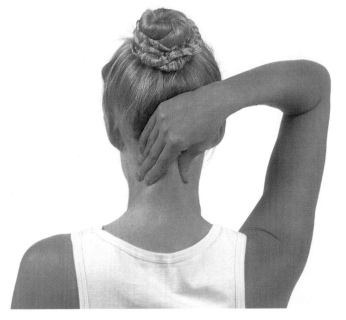

if your body calls out for some physical work to relieve aching, tired muscles.

Many activities inevitably lead to tensions in one part of the body or another, and regular quick massages can help both to ease these tensions and to prevent more chronic aches and pains, or even injury. At any time of the day a short self-massage can help you to feel revitalized and full of energy, and it will reduce the impact of stresses, both physical and mental. So, the next time you are feeling stiff, aching or just completely jaded, follow these simple techniques and put your hands to work to de-stress your whole system – and look and feel younger at the same time!

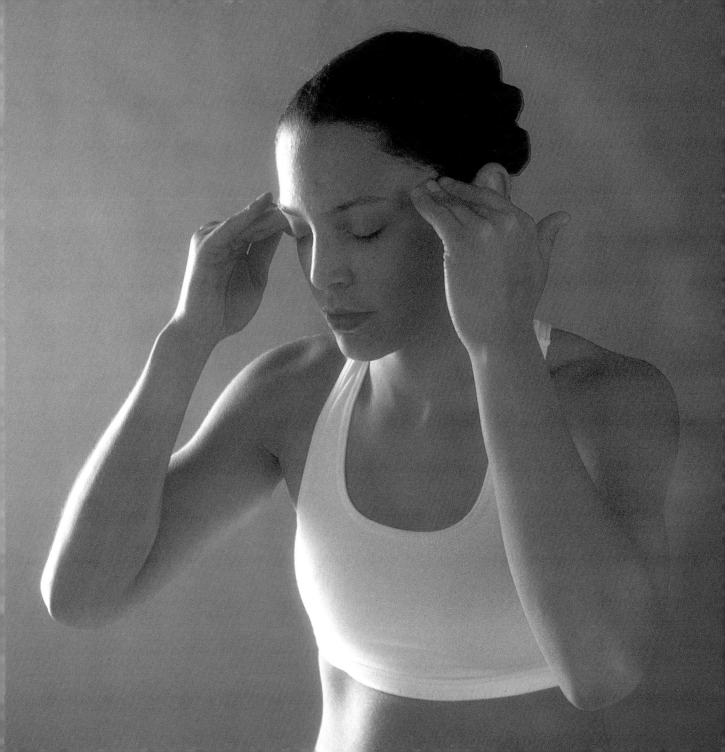

HAND TONIC

Your hands are among the most overworked parts of your body. For some people, such as keyboard operators, machinists and musicians, their hands are not only essential for their livelihoods but they may easily become strained through extended use. Repetitive strain injury may not yet have been fully recognized by the courts in all countries, but it is well-known both by the medical profession and by the workers who suffer its symptoms. Apart from regular breaks in repeated movement actions, self-massage of the hands and fingers can be of tremendous value. Swap hands with each massage technique.

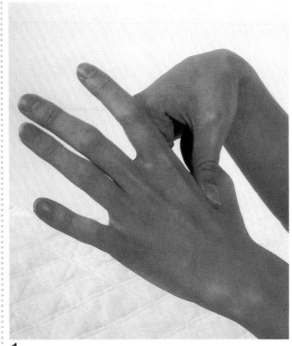

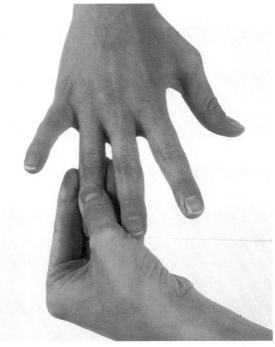

1 To release stored tensions and improve circulation, start by squeezing between each finger in turn with the thumb and index finger of the other hand.

2 Make a rolling movement on each finger, working from the knuckle to the fingertip with firm pressure from the fingers and thumb of the other hand.

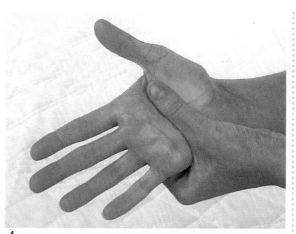

4 Finally, make a firm circling motion with one thumb on the palm of the other hand. This both squeezes and stretches taut, contracted muscles, and should be a fairly deep action; if done too lightly, it is merely ticklish.

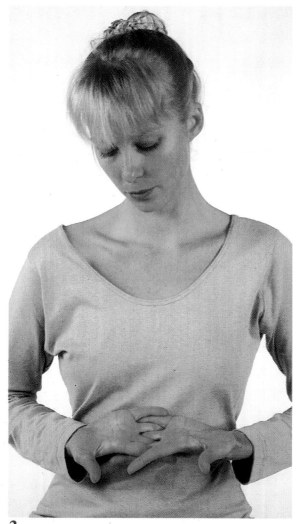

3 Stretch each finger, with a gentle pull to stretch out the tendons that tend to tighten with tension. It is not the intention to "crack" the fingers. Then interlock your fingers and stretch your palms.

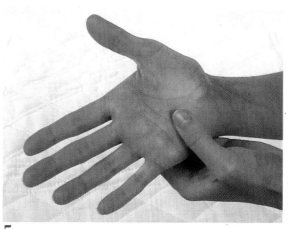

5 Work steadily all over the palm, maintaining a firm pressure the whole time.

TENSE NECK EASER

Aching, tense muscles are undoubtedly most usually experienced in the neck and shoulders. As you get tired, your posture tends to droop and the rounded shape makes your shoulders ache even more. Although it is most relaxing to lie down and have someone else massage them, self-massage of the shoulders and neck can be done anywhere, and without the need to get undressed. Release mounting tension in these areas before your shoulders become permanently hunched up around your ears.

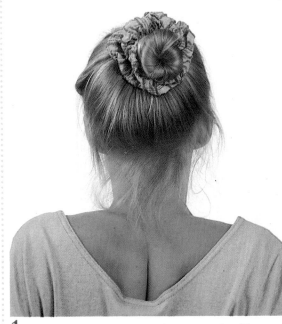

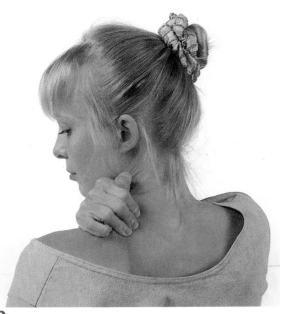

1 A simple movement is to shrug your shoulders, exaggerating their contraction by lifting them up as far as possible and then letting them drop down and relax completely. This is a form of massage that does not even involve using your hands.

2 One of the best massage techniques for removing waste matter from tired muscles and getting fresh, oxygenated blood into them, is kneading. You can do this to yourself – if the arm you are using starts to ache, rest a moment before continuing. Firmly grip your opposite shoulder with your hand and use a squeezing motion to loosen the tension.

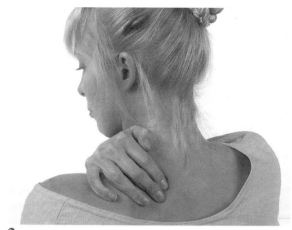

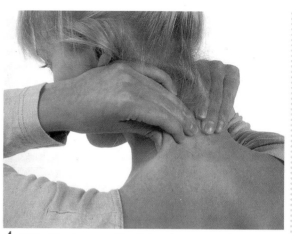

3 Move slowly along the shoulder, squeezing firmly several times. Repeat on the other side, using the opposite hand.

4 With the fingers of both hands, grip the back of the neck and squeeze in a circular motion to help to relax the muscles leading up either side of the neck.

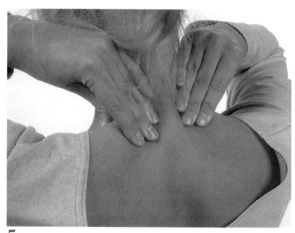

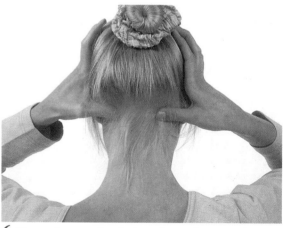

5 Work up as far as the base of the skull, and down again to the shoulders.

6 To work more deeply into the neck, move the thumbs in a circular movement across the neck and right up into the base of the skull. You will feel the bone as you apply moderate pressure.

TONIC FOR ACHING LEGS

Many people such as sales assistants (and indeed shoppers), teachers and hotel receptionists spend far too long each day standing still, or barely moving. Numerous occupations create real problems for circulation in our legs, which can lead to tired, aching limbs, swollen ankles or cramp. It is, of course, essential for people whose jobs involve a lot of standing to try and move their legs at other times, but a quick self-massage at the end of the day can help considerably in reducing stiffness and sluggishness of blood flow in the legs.

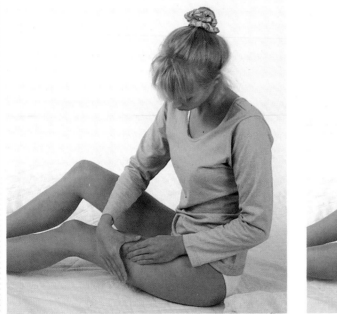

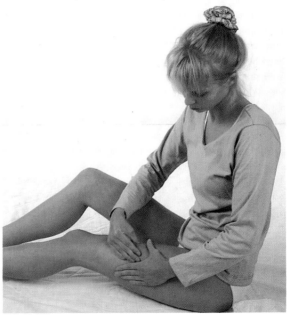

1 Start a leg massage by working on the thighs, so that any fluid retention in the calves will have somewhere to go as the upper leg relaxes. Using both hands, knead one thigh at a time, by squeezing between the fingers and thumb.

2 Squeeze with each hand alternately for the best effect, working from the knee to the hip and back. Repeat on the other thigh.

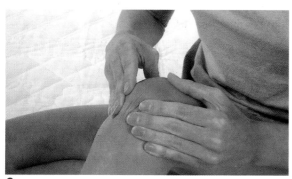

3 Around the knees, do a similar kneading action, but just using the fingers for a lighter effect and working in smaller circles.

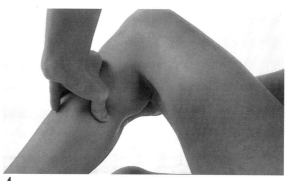

4 Bend your leg, and if possible raise the foot on to a chair or handy ledge. With your thumbs, work on the back of each calf with a circular, kneading action.

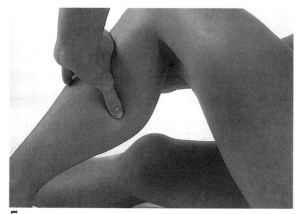

5 Repeat a few times, each time working from the ankle up the leg to the knee.

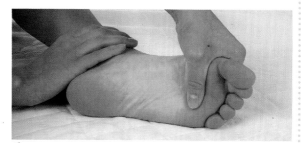

6 Squeeze the foot, loosening up the muscles and gently stretching the arch.

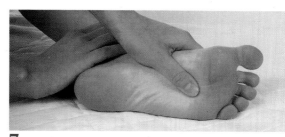

7 Use firm pressure with your thumb to stretch the foot. Repeat on the other foot.

INSTANT REVITALIZER

Do you find that you always run out of steam by 11 o'clock? Or by 4 o'clock?
Have you got to be bright and alert for a meeting, a long drive, picking up the kids or going
to a party? At any time of the day your energy can flag. Give yourself an instant "waker-upper"
with this simple yet effective routine.

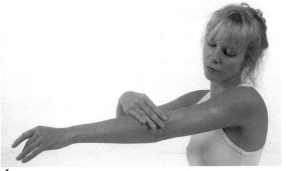

1 Do a kneading action on the arms, working rapidly from the wrist to the shoulder and back again with a firm squeezing movement.

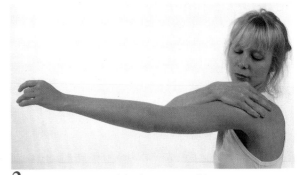

2 Knead more quickly than normal in massage, to invigorate each arm and shoulder in turn.

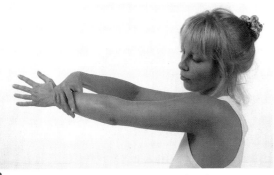

3 Then rub swiftly up the outside of each arm to stimulate the circulation.

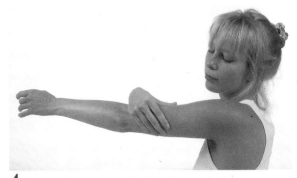

4 Repeat in an upwards direction each time to encourage blood flow back to the heart.

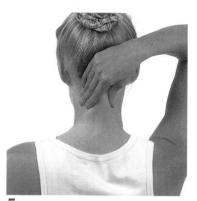

5 With the fingers and thumb of one hand, firmly squeeze the neck muscles using a circular motion.

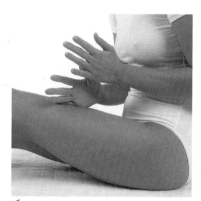

6 With the outside edge of the hands lightly hack on the front of each thigh, using a rapid motion.

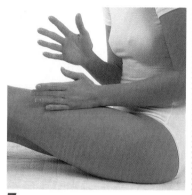

7 Do not try to karate-chop the thighs – the hands should spring up from the muscles.

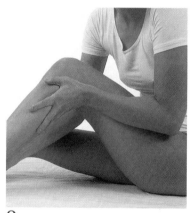

8 Next rub the calves vigorously to loosen them and get the blood moving. If possible, do this with the legs bent.

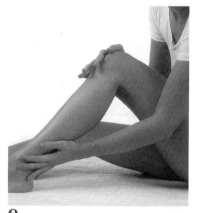

9 Always work from the ankles to the knee, using alternate hands.

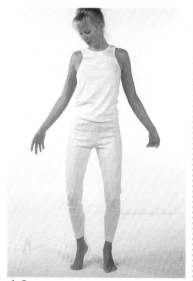

10 Finally, stand up and shake your whole body, to let go of any stiffness and tensions.

HEAD REVITALIZER

Almost everyone at some time or another suffers from headaches. They can have a multitude of causes, such as spending too much time in front of a VDU, anxiety, insomnia, fatigue or sinus congestion. However, the most common cause is from tension after periods of stress. Use this simple self-massage sequence to help ease headaches, whatever their cause. You can also use it any any time during the day to increase your vitality and help you to focus your mind.

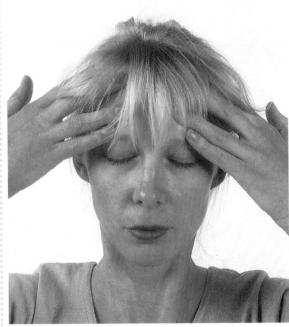

1 Use small, circling movements with the fingers, working steadily from the forehead down around the temples and over the cheeks.

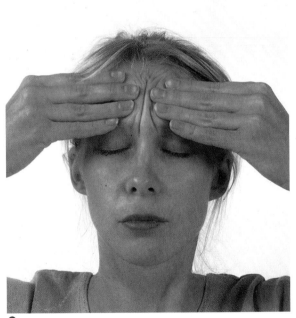

2 Use firm pressure and work slowly to ease tensions out of all the facial muscles.

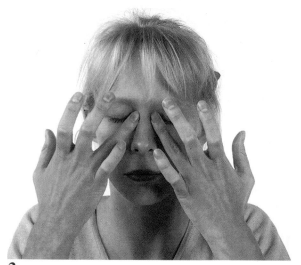

3 Use your fingers to gently press around the eye socket, by your nose.

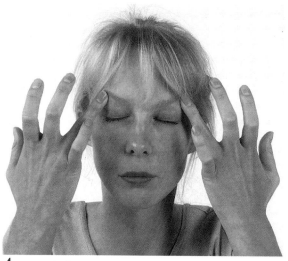

4 Smooth firmly, around the arc of your eye socket beneath your brow bone.

◀ **5** Work across the cheeks and along each side of the nose, then move out to the jaw line where a lot of tension is held. Try not to pull downwards on the skin – let the circling movements help to smooth the stresses away and gently lift the face as you work.

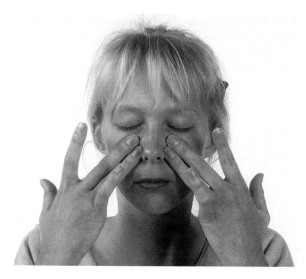

CHEST AND ABDOMEN RELEASER

The front of your body is an area where emotional tension is often stored; bottling up your feelings can create tight muscles across your chest or in your abdomen. Massage treatments on these areas often trigger the release of deep-seated emotions, and need a skilled, sensitive approach. Self-massage is, however, very helpful, both in easing tense muscles and also in helping to recognize where stored tensions lie. Being aware of the effects of stress is the first step towards letting go of it. Chest muscles can of course simply ache through unaccustomed exercise, and this simple sequence will help.

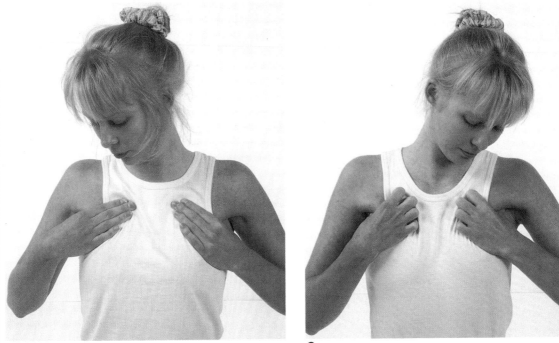

1 Using the thumb and fingers, take a good grip of the pectoral muscles, leading from the chest towards the shoulder, and knead them firmly.

2 Be careful if you have any tenderness in the lymph glands under the armpits; women should also go gently if they have tender, swollen breasts, for example when pre-menstrual.

▼ **3** Using a couple of fingers feel in between the ribs for the intercostal muscles, and work firmly along between each rib moving the fingers in tiny circles, repeating on each side.

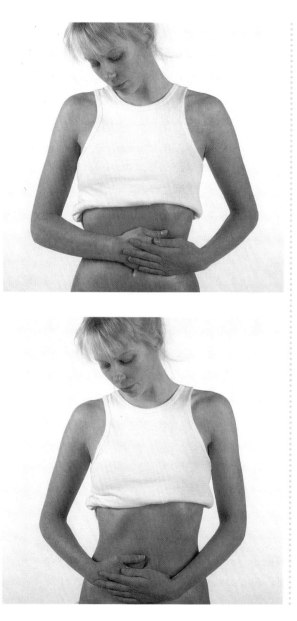

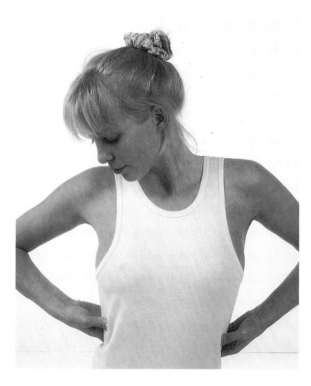

▶ **4** *Top right:* Place your hands on your abdomen, and work around *slowly* in a clockwise direction. If comfortable, repeat a couple of times with increasing pressure; ease off if this becomes painful.

▶ **5** By moving in this direction you encourage digestive and bowel action.

Shiatsu DoIn Exercises

In Shiatsu the term "DoIn" literally means "self-massage" and involves a combination of different techniques which stimulate pressure points along the meridians to improve the circulation and flow of Ki throughout the body. The following exercises can be used not only to revitalize tired muscles and low spirits, but also to relieve a stiff, tensed body and a stressed mind. Starting your day with a DoIn session will awaken your body and mind and help you feel refreshed and ready for the coming day. Repeating the routine in the evening before you go to bed will be physically and mentally relaxing and encourage a deep, peaceful night's sleep. Keep a natural posture and breathing throughout the exercises and try to maintain an empty mind, free from any disturbing thoughts and feelings.

Preparation

Prepare yourself by gently shaking out your body. Shake your arms and hands to help release any tension in your upper body. Gently shake out your legs and feet as well. Place your feet shoulder-width apart and unlock your knees. Straighten your back to allow better energy flow, relax your shoulders and close your eyes. Take a minute to focus internally and get in touch with how you and your body feel before starting the DoIn routine. Become aware of any areas that might be in discomfort and try to empty your mind of disturbing or distracting thoughts.

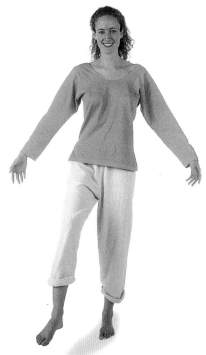

Head and face

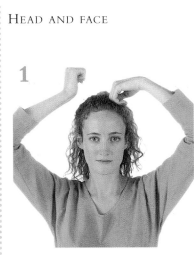

Open your eyes and make a loose fist with both hands. Keep your wrists relaxed and gently start to tap the top of your head.

2

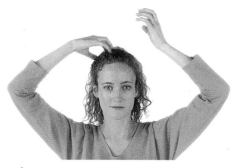

Adjust the percussion pressure as needed and use your fingertips or the palm of your hand for lighter stimulation. Slowly work your way all around the head, covering the sides, front and back. This exercise will wake up your brain and stimulate blood circulation, which will be beneficial for your mental focus and concentration as well as the quality of your hair.

3

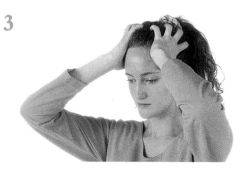

Pull your fingers through your hair a few times, stimulating the Bladder and Gall Bladder meridians running across the top and side of your head.

4

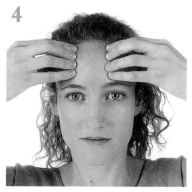

Place your fingers on your forehead, apply a little pressure and stroke outwards from the centre to the temples. Repeat this three times.

5

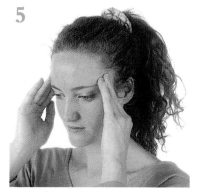

Bring your fingers to your temples. Drop your elbows, relax your shoulders and gently massage your temples, using small circular movements. This can prevent and relieve headaches.

6

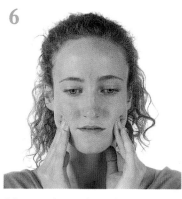

Massage down the sides of your face to the jaw.

7

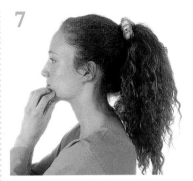

Squeeze along the jawbone, working outwards from the centre. This is a very good technique for relaxation and for stimulating the salivary glands.

8

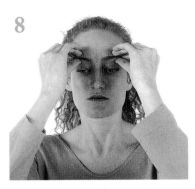

Using your index finger and thumb, squeeze your eyebrows starting from the centre line and moving laterally, three times.

9

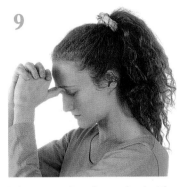

Bring your thumbs to the inside of the eyebrows. Allow the weight of your head to rest on your thumbs. This helps clear headaches and ease sinus problems.

10

With your index finger and thumb, pinch the bridge of the nose and the corners of the eyes. This point is the first one on the Bladder meridian and is called *Jing Ming*, meaning "Eye's Clarity". The name reflects the energetic function of this point on the eyes and vision. It opens and brightens your eyes, clears your vision and will be especially helpful when your eyes are tired.

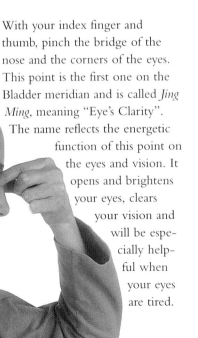

11

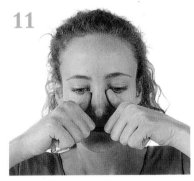

Clench your fingers and apply your thumbs to the sides of your nose. Breathe in as you quickly stroke down the side of your nose. This will help clear your sinuses and release any nasal congestion. Repeat three times.

NECK

Using one hand, place the palm across the back of
your neck and firmly massage in a squeezing motion.
This will increase the flow of blood and Ki to the
area, release stagnation and remove waste products,
such as lactic acid.

1

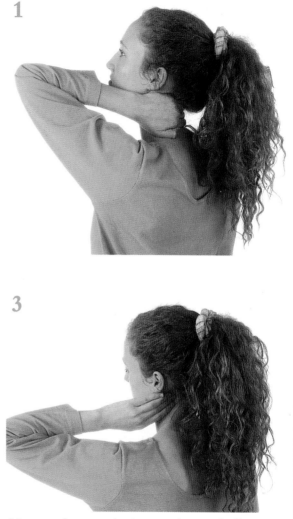

2

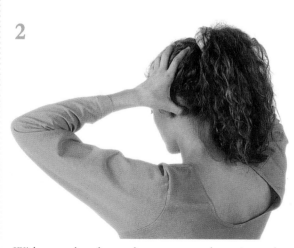

With your thumbs, apply pressure to the point at the
base of the skull, directing the pressure upwards against
the skull.

3

Use your fingers and rub across the muscle fibres at
the base of the skull. This will release the muscles and
tendons in the area and help relieve headaches and
shoulder pain.

SHOULDERS, ARMS AND HANDS

After doing these exercises shake out your arms. Allow them to relax and compare the feeling in them. Your right arm probably feels lighter, more vital and expanded compared to the left. This shows that there is a better energy flow in your right arm. Repeat the same techniques on your left arm and hand and then compare them again.

1

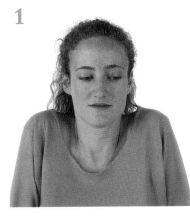

Lift your shoulders up and breathe in. Breathe out, letting your shoulders drop and relax. Repeat.

2

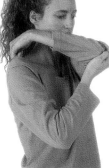

Support your left elbow and with a loose fist tap across your shoulder.

3

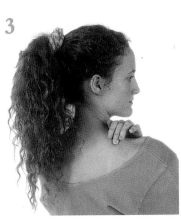

Press your middle finger into the shoulder's highest point, known as the "Shoulder Well".

Caution *Do not use in pregnancy.*

4

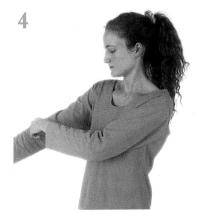

Straighten your arm, open your palm and tap down the inside of your arm from the shoulder to the open hand. This stimulates the energy flow of the Lung, Heart Governor and Heart meridians.

5

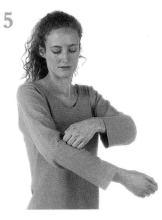

Turn your arm over and tap up the back of your arm, from the hand to the shoulders. This stimulates the meridians for the Large Intestine, Triple Heater and Small Intestine. Repeat three times.

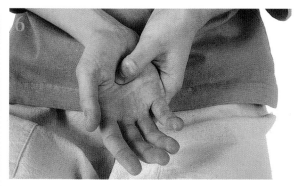

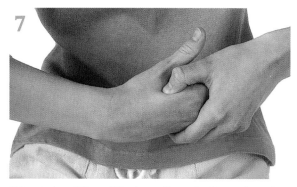

Use your left thumb to work through your right hand, gently massaging the centre of your palm to stimulate the point there, also known as "Palace of Anxiety". This will relieve general tension and revitalize you physically, mentally and spiritually.

Stimulating "Great Eliminator" on the Large Intestine meridian, in the web between the index finger and the thumb, will help relieve headaches and can also be used to treat constipation or diarrhoea. Good for general health and well-being.

Caution *Sometimes used in childbirth to speed up labour; do not use during pregnancy.*

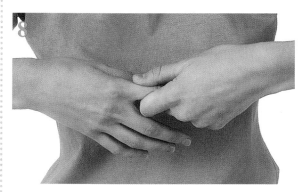

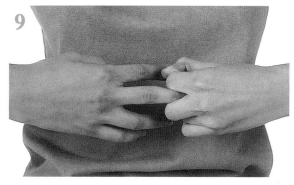

Squeeze and massage the joints of each finger using your index finger and thumb.

Pulling out the fingers will stimulate the starting and end points of all the meridians. This is a great way to release any stress and tension in your hands and will help prevent arthritis as well as improve flexibility in the joints.

CHEST, ABDOMEN AND LOWER BACK

1

Open up your chest, and using either a loose fist or flat hands for comfort, tap across your chest, above and around the breasts and across your ribs. This will stimulate your lungs, enhance and strengthen your respiratory system and improve your blood and Ki circulation. Children love this exercise. It is wonderful for releasing tension in your chest, usually brings a smile to your face and will support you in expressing your inner thoughts and feelings.

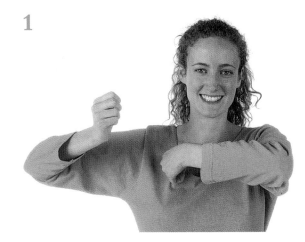

2

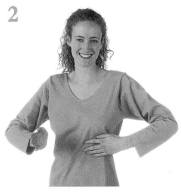

Take a deep breath in as you open your chest again; on the out breath tap your chest and make an "Ahhh…" sound.

3

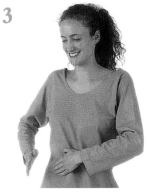

Proceed further down towards your abdomen, and with open hands gently tap around your abdomen in a clockwise direction, moving down on the left side and up on the right. This follows the flow of circulation and digestion. Do this for about a minute.

4

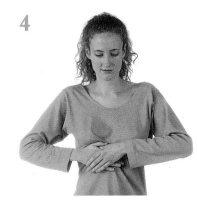

Place one hand on top of the other and make the same circular motion around your abdomen for another minute.

5

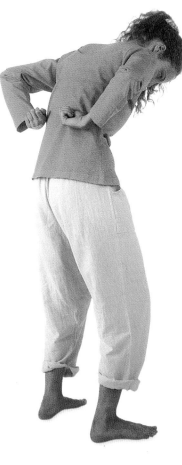

6

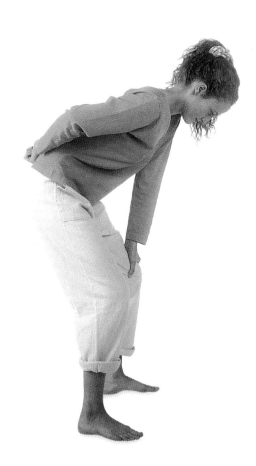

Place your hands on your back, just below your ribcage. This is the area of your kidneys. Start to rub the area until you feel some warmth building up underneath your hands and then proceed to tap the area gently using a loose fist. This will stimulate your Kidney energy responsible for your vitality and also for warming your body.

Lean forward and place one hand on your knee. Using the back of your other hand, tap across the sacrum bone at the base of your spine. This will activate your nervous system and send energy vibrations up the spine to your head and brain, bringing clarity to your mental processes.

LEGS

Proceed from the sacrum to your hips and buttocks. Tapping this area will help release muscle tension and stimulate your digestive and elimination organs.

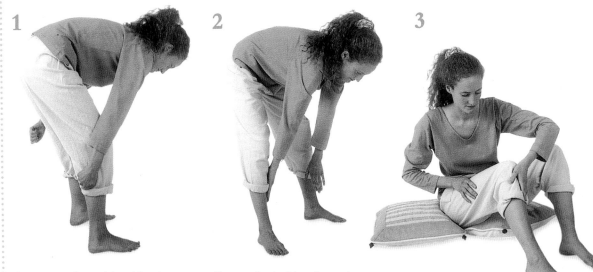

1

Open your feet a bit wider, keep your knees slightly bent and tap down the backs of your legs from your buttocks to your heels, following the flow of energy in your Bladder meridian.

2

Tap up the inside of your legs from the ankles to the groin area, stimulating your Liver and Spleen meridians. Tap down the outside of your legs to stimulate your Gall Bladder meridian and come up the inside of your legs again. Finally tap down the fronts of your legs, slightly outside the big quadriceps muscle, activating your Stomach meridian. Tap all the way down to the fronts of your ankles and then come back up the inside of your legs.

3

To find the pressure point on the Stomach meridian that is good ofr general well-being and tired legs, sit down on the floor, and measure four finger widths down from the patella (knee-cap) on the outside of your leg, along the tibia bone. Place your thumb on the point and apply pressure.

FEET 1

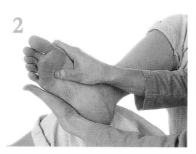

Sit on the floor, take your right foot in your hands and circle it from the ankle to mobilize the joint generally.

On the dorsal part of your foot, between the big toe and the second toe is the point called "Big Rush", a very good point to stimulate if you experience abdominal spasm and cramps.
Caution *Do not use this point during pregnancy.*

3

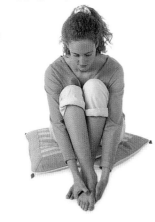

2

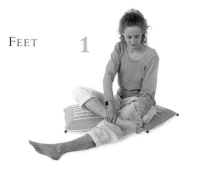

Massage the sole of your foot using your thumbs. About one-third of the distance from the base of the second toe to the back of your heel, you will find "Gushing Spring". The name suggests this point's fresh and active energy and stimulating it with pressure will have a revitalizing effect upon your whole system. Give the whole foot an invigorating rub.

Take hold of your ankle with both hands and shake out your foot. Repeat the same sequence with your left foot.

COMPLETION

After having worked through your whole body, stand up and gently shake out again. Place your feet shoulder-width apart and bend your knees slightly. Imagine a string through your spine, from the tail bone to the top of your head. Stretch the string and feel your spine straighten up to allow for better Ki flow. Close your eyes for a moment and see how you feel after your DoIn session. Try to remember how you felt at the beginning and compare that with the sensation you have now.

Open your eyes again and take a series of deep, slow breaths to calm your mind.

4

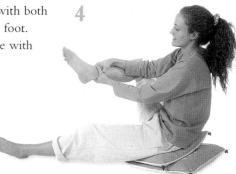

MASSAGE WITH A PARTNER

PROBABLY THE BEST WAY to improve and deepen a relationship is to increase caring physical contact, and massage is an ideal approach. The ability to ease tensions and deeply relax your partner is a very satisfying form of giving. Helping someone to release tension and feel better does not have to be limited to your life partner of course; there are other members of the family, friends or colleagues who can all be helped in this way, and a better rapport will be developed with them too.

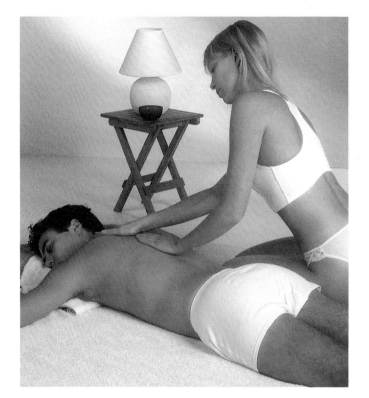

Being massaged by someone else does mean that you can let go of your muscles more completely. It does require an amount of trust, and if you are massaging a person you do not know too well, do be sensitive to this. Massage practitioners are well aware that they are being given permission to make a deep contact with their clients, which is quite a privilege.

Take a few moments to make sure that you have created the right environment for a beneficial and relaxing massage. Check that the person is warm and comfortable, and that you have easy access to the part needing massage. Do not press harder than is comfortable for your partner and take care never to inflict pain.

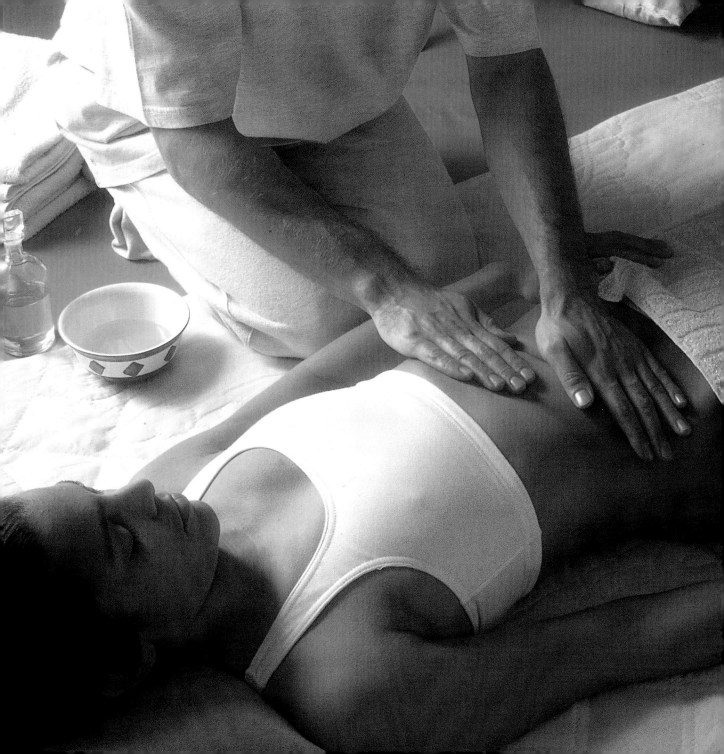

HEADACHE AND TENSION RELIEVER

One of the most common symptoms people experience when they get stressed is a tension headache; for some, this can become almost a daily pattern and may lead to migraine attacks. Any treatment should be given at the earliest stage, and massage is no exception. Just a few minutes of soothing strokes can prevent major muscle spasm and head pain.

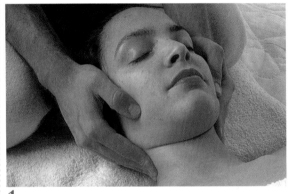

1 Ideally have the person lying down with the head in your lap, or on a cushion, while you kneel or sit just behind them.

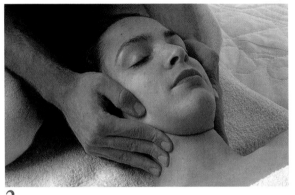

2 Using your fingertips, make alternating circles on the muscles either side of the neck.

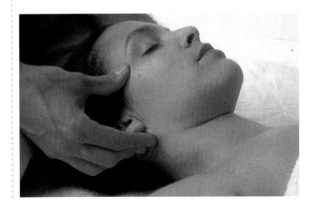

◄ **3** Continue circling, this time with both hands working at the same time, around the side of the head and behind the ears.

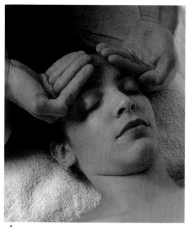

4 Smooth tension away from the temples with the backs or sides of your hands, in a stroking motion.

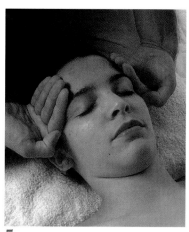

5 Gently draw the hands outwards across the forehead to soothe away worry lines.

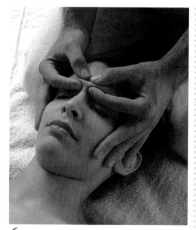

6 Pinch and squeeze along the line of the eyebrows, reducing pressure as you work outwards.

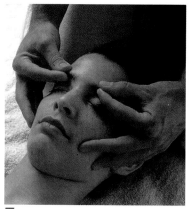

7 These muscles may be quite tender, so try not to apply too much pressure.

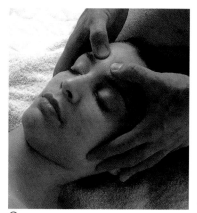

8 With your thumbs, use steady but firm pressure on the forehead, working outwards from between the eyebrows.

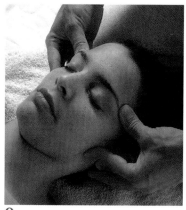

9 Work across the brow to the hair line. This also covers many acupressure points, and will release blocked energy.

SLEEP-ENHANCING FACIAL SOOTHER

If your partner has frequent problems with sleeping, or simply carries a lot of tension around in the facial muscles, this facial soother might be the answer. So why not treat your partner to this ten-minute programme at bedtime? Apart from being great for relaxation, working on these muscles will smooth out worry lines and re-invigorate the face, making your partner look years younger – don't forget to request a facial massage for yourself in return!

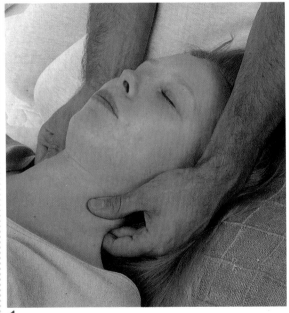

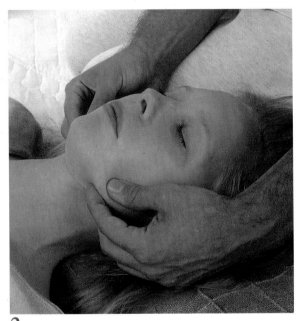

1 Kneeling behind the head, place both your hands under your partner's neck. Pull on the neck muscles *gently*, creating a little traction to stretch out the neck and head.

2 With your fingertips make small circling movements along the jawline and over the cheeks. Use firm pressure, but as with all massage, avoid causing any discomfort. Try to work symmetrically, both hands working at the same time.

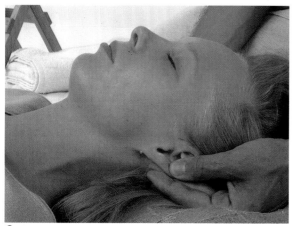

3 Pull gently with the fingertips and stretch the ears, working around from the earlobes to the top of the ears and back again.

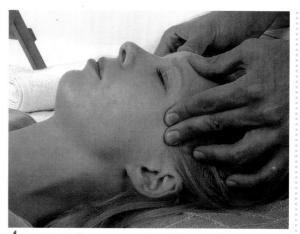

4 Apply circling movements with your fingers or thumbs on the temples and forehead, easing the pressure as you work up the temples.

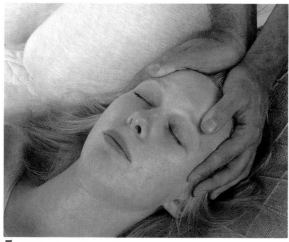

5 With the palms of your hands, smooth across the forehead, easing out tension and worry lines.

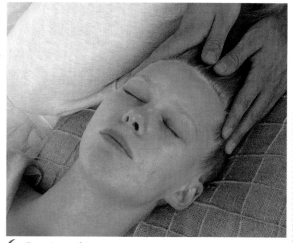

6 Continue this movement, but now working your hands towards you, and extend it by stroking up into the hair to complete the sequence.

NECK AND SHOULDER RELIEVER

Most people feel tension in their neck or shoulders at times; when you describe others – or yourself – as being uptight, it is indeed these very areas that are holding all the stresses. People who have a strong sense of responsibility are often very tense in this area, as they metaphorically "carry the world on their shoulders". Often tension in the shoulders is reflected in tight muscles lower down the back, and for a deeper effect, use the following back massage as well as the techniques described here. The muscle that takes the main brunt of tension in the shoulder is the trapezius; this is the muscle that stands out on either side when you shrug your shoulders, and it connects right up into the neck and down to the middle of the back. Lifting weights, gardening, bending over papers and driving are typical activities that tighten the trapezius; one of the best ways to loosen it is by kneading.

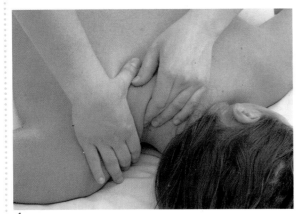

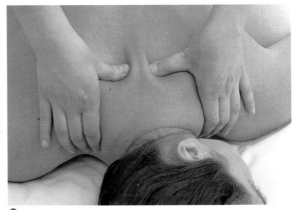

1 This technique takes a little time to master but is well worth the effort. Place both hands on the opposite shoulder, and with alternate hands squeeze your fingers and thumb together. Do not pinch, but roll the fingers over the thumb. Repeat by moving to the other side, again working on the shoulder away from your body. Ideally, get your partner to turn his or her head towards you each time, so that your fingers do not knock into the chin while kneading.

2 Having worked on each shoulder in turn, now work on both together. Place your thumbs on either side of the spine on the upper back, with the rest of each hand over each shoulder. Squeeze your fingers and thumbs together, rolling the flesh between them.

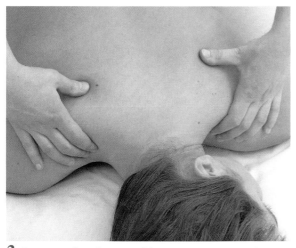

3 Let your thumbs smoothly move out across the shoulder muscles.

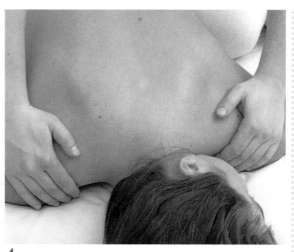

4 Release the pressure of the thumbs and stretch the blades outwards with the hands.

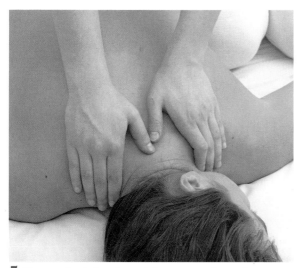

5 Return both hands to the centre and get the thumbs in position to repeat.

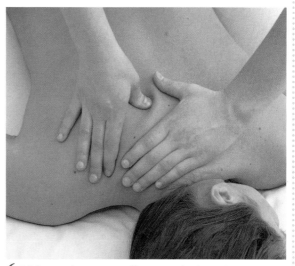

6 If the neck is very stiff, repeat the kneading, applying firmer pressure with the thumbs.

TENSION AND BACKACHE RELIEVER

The back is where most of our physical aches and pains are generally located; more days are lost off work each year through back problems than all other parts of the body put together. It is a good area to massage, with broad, relaxing movements that cannot easily be carried out elsewhere. People can unwind, lying face down, and you may find your partner is asleep by the time you finish!

All the basic strokes are applicable to working on the back, and students on a massage course often learn many of the movements here first. Remember, if you need to apply more pressure with any movement, simply lean your whole body into the action. Try not to tense your fingers or hands as this will make the action less comfortable rather than deeper.

Apply oil smoothly to the back, remembering to put it on to your own hands before spreading it on your partner's skin, in order to warm the oil. Use enough to allow your hands to move easily over the skin without dragging, but avoid making your partner look like a professional wrestler.

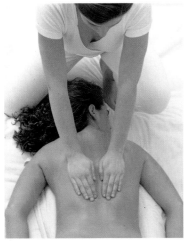

1 The best initial movement is effleurage. Sit or kneel at the head end and place your hands on the back, with the thumbs close to, but not on, the spine.

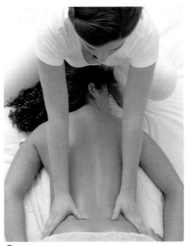

2 Steadily lean forward and glide your hands down the back, keeping a steady pressure all the way.

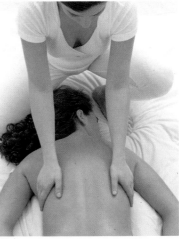

3 Maintaining the same pressure and slow pace, take your hands out to the side and bring them back up to the shoulders.

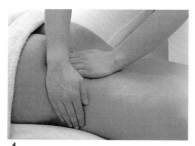

4 Kneeling at the side, place your hands on the other side of the back and move them steadily in a circular motion, using overlapping circles to work up and down the back. Move to the other side and repeat the circling technique.

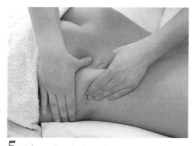

5 Place both hands on the opposite side of the back and use a squeezing motion, with alternate hands, to create a kneading effect.

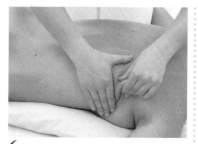

6 The fingers and thumbs of each hand work towards each other in a kind of pinching movement, the fingers rolling over the top of the thumbs. Repeat on the other side.

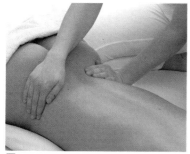

7 With one hand on the side of the back nearest you, and the other hand on the opposite side, push the hands towards and then past each other to reverse their position. This makes a wringing effect as they squeeze the muscles against the spine. Move up and down the back slowly and firmly.

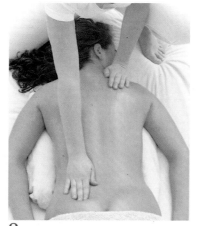

8 Place your hands centrally on the back and then push them away from each other, leaning forward to maintain an even pressure during this stretch.

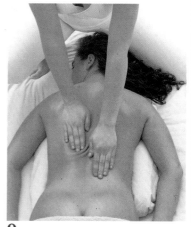

9 Reverse the movements to create a wringing effect as the hands pass each other before stretching out the back as they push apart.

LOWER BACK RELAXER

A classic area for storing and feeling tension is in the lumbar part of the back, where it curves backwards towards the pelvis. Incorrect posture, long periods of sitting or standing, and lifting things awkwardly are just some of the many causes that can all aggravate lower back discomfort. If your partner suffers from twinges in this area, a regular massage will stretch and relax the back, and help to prevent more serious pains or injury.

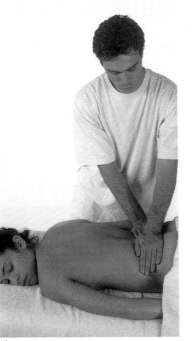

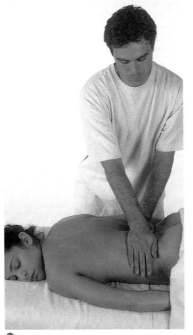

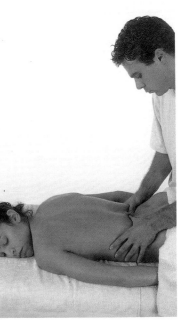

1 Standing or kneeling to the side, place your hands on the opposite side of the person's back and pull them towards you firmly and alternately.

2 Overlap the hands to create an effect like bandaging – but much more soothing.

3 Using your thumbs, make circling movements over the lower back. Use a steady, even pressure, leaning with your body, but do not press on the spine.

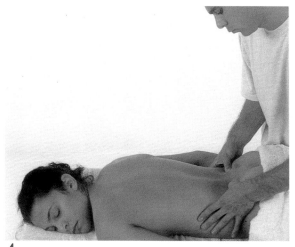

4 Stretch the lower back muscles by gliding the thumbs firmly up either side several times.

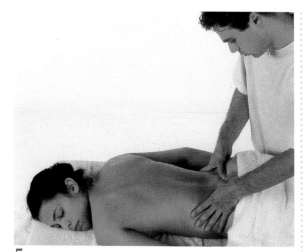

5 Press in steadily with both thumbs just on either side of the spine, working slowly up it.

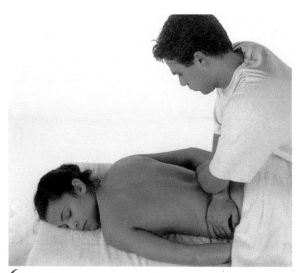

6 Stretch across the lower back with crossed hands moving away from each other, to ease taut muscles.

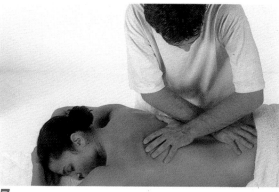

7 Push the hands apart and stretch the whole back.

CAUTION: Do not put any pressure on the spine itself, and ease off if it feels uncomfortable.

LEG ENERGIZER

Exercise, or lack of it, long hours of standing or sitting can all lead to stiff, aching leg muscles.
If massaging the whole body, carry on from the back by working on the backs of the legs before
getting your partner to turn over and settle comfortably again for the front.

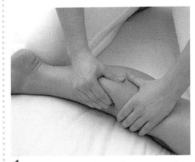

1 Knead the calves; do not apply too much pressure.

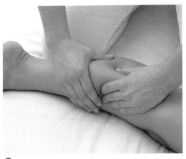

2 If possible work up and down on the inside of the calf and then on the outside, as the muscle "splits" into two distinct halves.

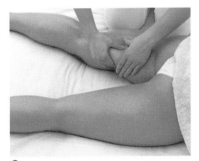

3 Knead the back of the thighs, working more to the outside to avoid the sensitive inner thigh.

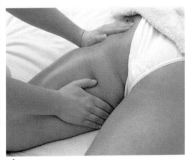

4 Firm pressure with the heel of the hand up the thigh will release tight muscles.

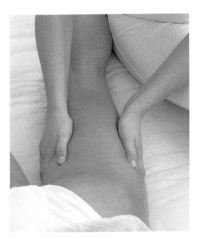

5 Stroke smoothly and steadily up the whole back of the leg, moving the blood flow back towards the heart and draining waste matter from the muscles.

CAUTION:
Never apply any pressure directly behind the knee and never put pressure on, or squeeze, varicose veins.

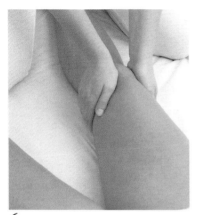

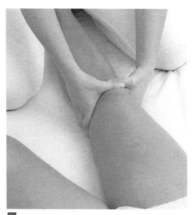

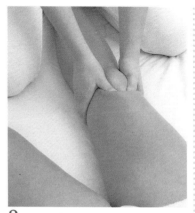

6 The front of the lower legs is mostly bone so avoid this area and move directly to the knees.

7 Make circling movements around the knees, with the thumbs. Do not put pressure directly on the kneecaps.

8 Bring the thumbs to the top of the knees and continue to circle around the edges of the kneecaps.

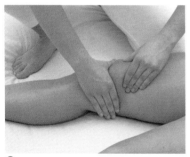

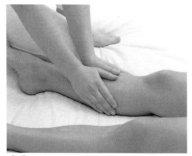

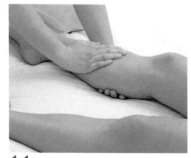

9 Kneading of the front of the thighs will help to release tight muscles and improve blood flow. Use each hand alternately, squeezing your fingers and thumb together without pinching; work more to the outside again, to avoid the sensitive inner thigh.

10 Stroke all the way up the front of the legs using both hands, always in an upwards motion back towards the heart to encourage blood and lymph drainage.

11 Lighter pressure, using the flat of the palm, may be more comfortable if the veins are at all prominent. Do *not* press on varicose veins or any area of inflammation.

INSTANT FOOT REVITALIZER

With really very little complaint, your feet carry you around all day long. When you compare the size of your feet with the rest of you, it is not surprising if they sometimes do feel tight or sore. Relieve tired, aching feet with a ten-minute massage, and let them feel like dancing again!

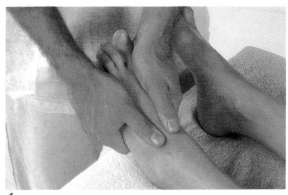

1 Hold the foot in your hands, with thumbs on top and fingers underneath.

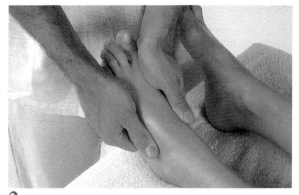

2 Gently stretch across the top of the foot; try to keep your fingers still while moving your thumbs.

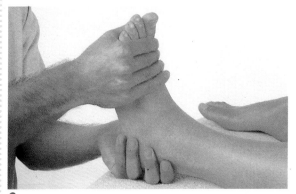

3 Flex the foot, pushing against the resistance to loosen the whole foot and ankle a little.

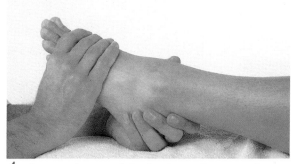

4 Then gently extend the foot, stretching it as far as is comfortable.

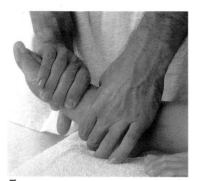

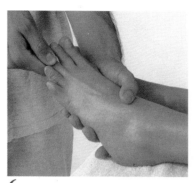

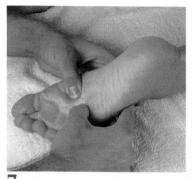

5 Twist the foot gently, using a wringing motion, in both directions to stretch the muscles in every way.

6 Hold one of the toes and give a squeeze and pulling action. Repeat for all the toes.

7 Circle over the sole firmly with your fingers, or thumbs if that is easier; make sure you do not tickle your partner.

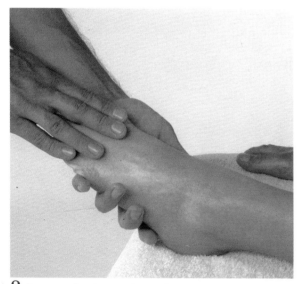

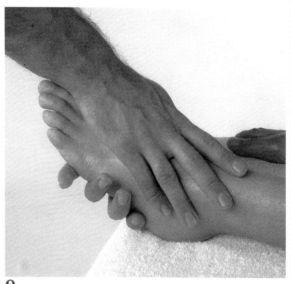

8 Support the foot with one hand and stroke the upper side with the other hand.

9 Smoothly stroke all the way from the toes to the ankle. Repeat all the actions on the other foot.

ARM AND HAND TONIC

More than any other part of your body, you use your hands and arms for all kinds of physical tasks – at work, for household chores or in leisure activities. As a result, they are often stiff and tense; a few simple massage techniques can help to shed the tensions and burdens of the day.

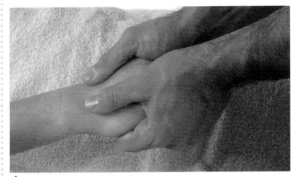

1 Kneel by your partner, who is lying face up. Hold your partner's hand, palm down, in both of your hands and with your thumbs apply a steady stretching motion across the back of the hand.

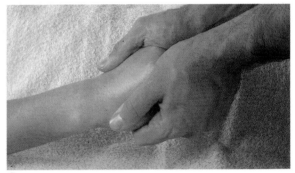

2 Repeat a few times, with a firm but comfortable pressure. Turn the hand over and use your thumbs to smooth and stretch the palm in a similar action.

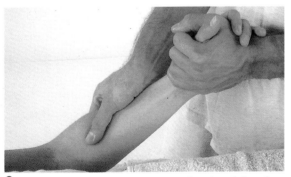

3 Squeeze the forearm, using your hand and thumb to work from the wrist towards the elbow.

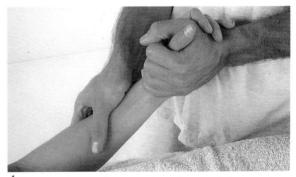

4 Repeat the motion, moving all around the arm to squeeze all the muscles.

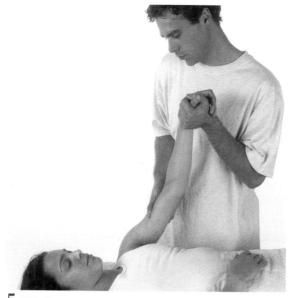

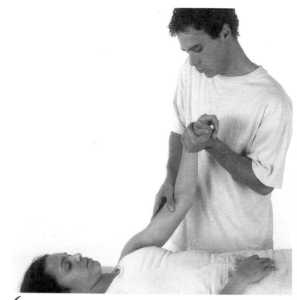

5 Lift the arm right up, and then use a similar squeezing movement to work down the upper arm, from the elbow to the shoulder.

6 Repeat, working all around the arm. Swap hands if necessary for a more comfortable action. Repeat all these movements on the other arm.

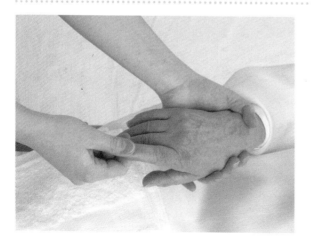

◀ Older people often find that their fingers are not as dextrous as they once were. As long as the joints are not inflamed or in a degenerated condition, a regular hand massage with gentle movements and finger stretches will aid continued flexibility.

TENSE ABDOMEN RELIEVER

Tension in the abdomen may reflect some physical discomfort, such as indigestion, constipation or menstrual cramp. Often, though, people hold their inner fears and anxieties in this area. If you bottle up your feelings, then you can become literally unable to digest stress, and abdominal spasm may occur. Try these movements, working slowly and just as deeply as feels comfortable to your partner.

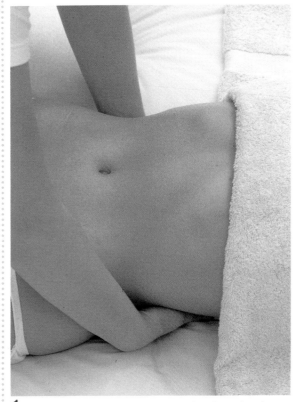

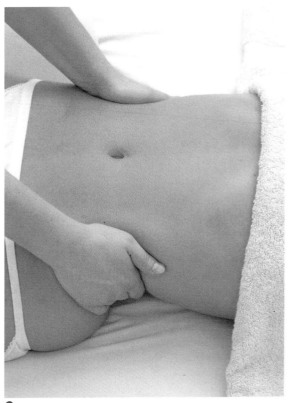

1 Kneeling by the side, slide your hands under the back to meet at the spine. Lift the body to arch the back before pulling your hands out towards the hips.

2 Firmly draw your hands over the waist and then gently glide them back to their original position to repeat the stroke.

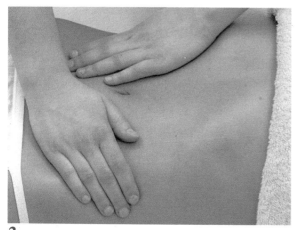

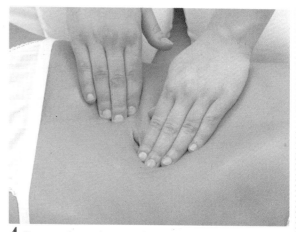

3 Placing your hands on the abdomen, move them around steadily in a clockwise direction (this follows the way in which the colon functions).

4 Repeat the action, working a little deeper by using your fingers if there is no discomfort.

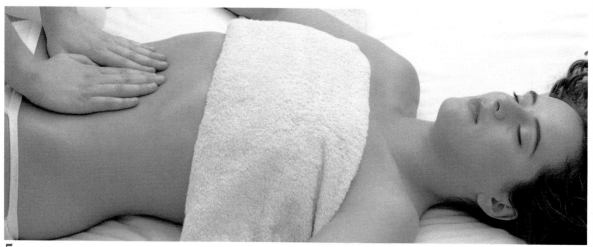

5 Place your hands on the abdomen, over the navel, and simply try to make your hands and arms as relaxed as possible. Focus calming thoughts down through your own body into your partner. You may be surprised at how effective this simple technique can be in helping to relax tense muscles.

TREATING STRESS AT YOUR DESK

The build-up of tension and pain in the neck and shoulders are common symptoms of today's pressured and stressful work environments. The following quick-and-easy Shiatsu routine is designed for the workplace and will give relief to the accumulating tension in the neck and shoulders.

TUNING IN

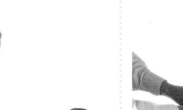

Have your partner sit on a chair with proper back support to encourage a straight spine. This will allow for better energy flow. Make contact with your partner's shoulders·and take a minute to tune in and see how your partner feels at this moment. Be aware of any tension your partner might hold in the shoulders and listen to the breathing.

KNEADING THE SHOULDERS

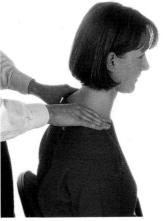

Grip and hold the trapezius muscles (the muscles of the shoulders and neck) on either side of the neck. Squeeze these muscles a few times, combining your thumbs and fingers in a rhythmic "kneading" action. There may be tension initially but this will slowly dissolve. Work within your partner's pain threshold.

LIFTING THE SHOULDERS

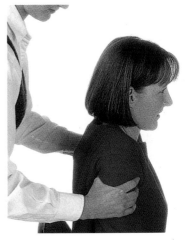

To encourage your partner to relax into the treatment, take a firm grip of their upper arms; ask your partner to breathe in as you lift the shoulders up and breathe out as you allow the shoulders to drop back down again. Repeat three times.

HACKING ACROSS THE SHOULDERS

Keep your own shoulders, wrists and hands relaxed and "soft". Use a gentle hacking action with the sides of your hands and move rhythmically across the shoulders and base of the neck. Increase the intensity and power of the hacking as the muscles relax and your partner's discomfort, if any, disappears.

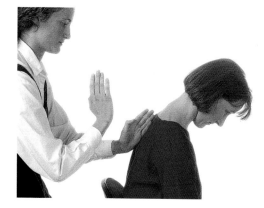

1

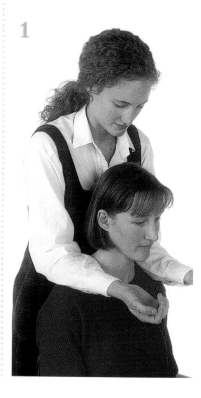

APPLYING PRESSURE TO THE SHOULDERS

Stand close to your partner for support. Place your forearms on the shoulders, and on the out-breath lean into your arms, applying perpendicular pressure downwards. Repeat three times.

Move slightly to the side. Place one hand in front and with the other thumb apply pressure to any points on top of the shoulder. Choose points you feel intuitively attracted to. These might feel sore and sensitive to start with, but as the muscle tissue gradually relaxes and the points open up, the pain will dissolve and warmth will spread across the shoulders.

2

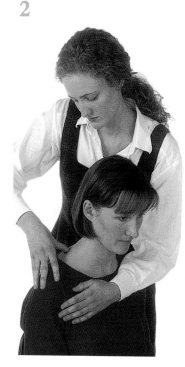

SHOULDER STRETCH

Take hold of your partner's elbow and stretch open the shoulder by bringing the elbow across the chest. With your forearm, lean into the shoulder to increase the stretch. Shoulders are more likely to become stiff when there are problems with the digestive system. This technique will open up the energy channels running over the shoulders – Gall Bladder, Large Intestine and Small Intestine – and stimulate the digestive system into balance.

Move yourself over to the other side and treat the other shoulder in the same way.

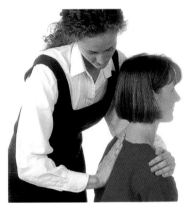

PALMING THE SPINE

Palm down your partner's spine to encourage an upright posture and stimulate the Bladder channel (affecting and calming the whole nervous system).

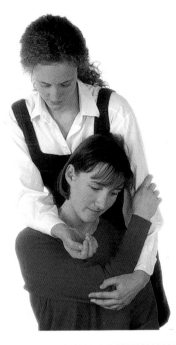

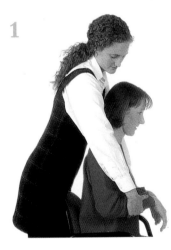

1

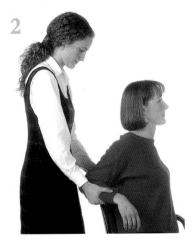

2

OPENING OF THE CHEST

Stand behind your partner and take hold of the lower arms.

Ask your partner to take a deep breath in; on the exhalation bring the elbows towards each other behind the back. Repeat three times. This will open up and expand the chest and encourage better breathing with improved posture.

SQUEEZING THE NECK

Stand at your partner's side. Ask your partner to relax and drop the head forward into your left hand. Hold the forehead until you feel your partner has given up control of the neck. Using the fingers and thumb of your right hand, gently squeeze the muscles of the neck, patiently working from top to bottom.

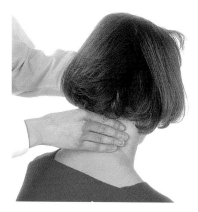

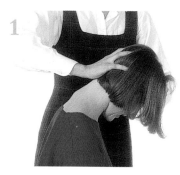

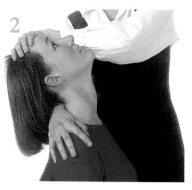

STRETCHING THE NECK

Keep your left hand on your partner's forehead and with your right hand support the neck into a forward stretch, opening up the back of the neck and the spine.

Place your right arm across your partner's shoulders. Apply a gentle lifting movement with your forearm as your left hand guides the head backwards on to your forearm. This will stretch the front of the neck.

Caution *The base of the skull and neck must always be supported by your forearm to prevent too strong a movement backwards, which could cause injury.*

COMPLETION

Support your partner's forehead with your left hand and bring the index finger and thumb of your right hand to the base of the skull. Imagine yourself "lifting" your partner from this position, stretching out the entire spine from sacrum to head. Ask your partner to close their eyes and hold the position for a minute, allowing your partner to feel the energy moving up and down the spine. Finish the treatment by slowly moving your hands away.

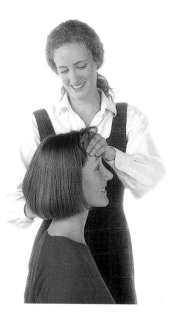

LIBIDO ENHANCER: SENSUAL MASSAGE

As well as releasing stresses and tensions from the muscles, massage is a wonderful way to enhance a relationship, by increasing caring, sharing touch. If your relationship seems to have got into a rut, and sexual energy is low, why not revitalize yourselves with some soothing massage strokes. It is important to take a little extra time to create the right environment, to make the whole experience a real treat – time for you both in a hurried world. Make the room extra warm, get your partner to be minimally clothed or to undress fully, and just be covered with warm towels, perhaps play some of your favourite, soothing music and have soft lighting or better still, work in candle light. Stroking movements should be the mainstay of a sensual massage. Use a little more oil than usual to help them flow more easily. At the end, your partner may of course just fall asleep.

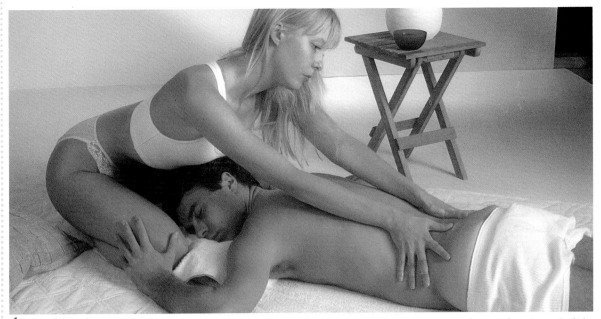

1 Effleurage is a classic stroking movement. Place your hands on either side of the spine, but not on it, and glide down the back. Move out to the sides and up the back again. Repeat several times.

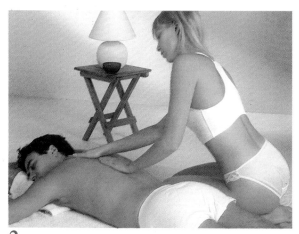

2 With a gentle motion, stroke down the centre of the back with one hand following the other smoothly, as if you were stroking a cat.

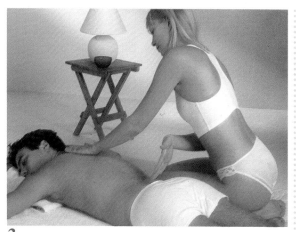

3 As one hand lifts off at the pelvis, start again with the other hand at the neck.

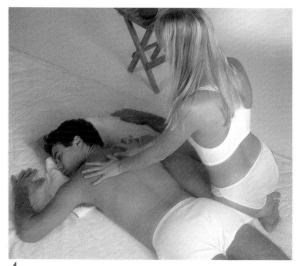

4 Place both your hands on the upper back and stroke outwards in a fan shape.

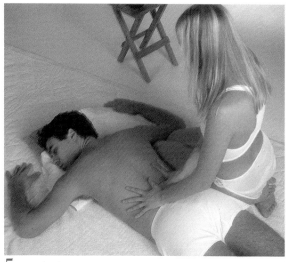

5 Work down the back, including the buttocks, using the fanning action.

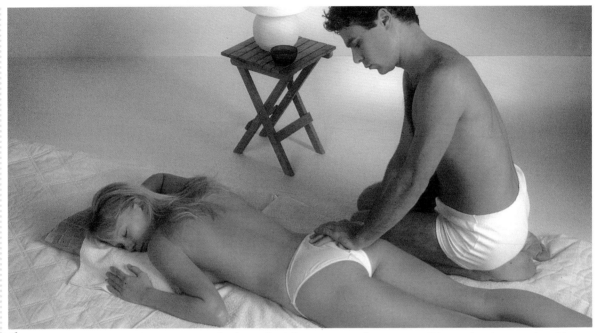

6 Use a firm, steady circling action on the buttocks. These are very large, powerful muscles that may be able to take a little more pressure if your partner desires, but avoid giving any discomfort.

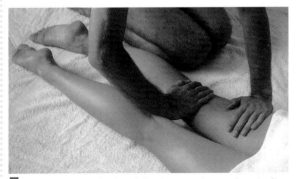

7 Stroke up the back of the legs, with one hand after the other in a smooth, flowing motion.

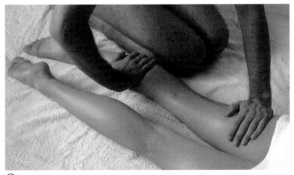

8 As one hand reaches the buttocks, start on the calf with the other to keep a steady rhythm.

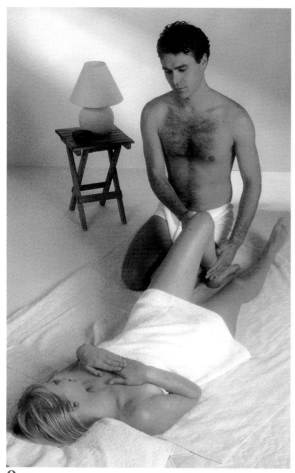

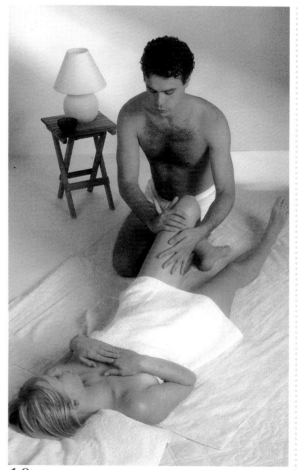

9 Turn your partner over and stroke up the front of the legs; having the leg bent helps the muscles relax.

10 Continue the movement, using both hands to stroke from the knees up the thighs.

11 Effleurage may also be used on the front of the body, kneeling from the head end. Be careful not to press in with your thumbs. All these movements should make for a truly sensual experience, and help to put your partner back in touch with his or her body – and maybe yours too.

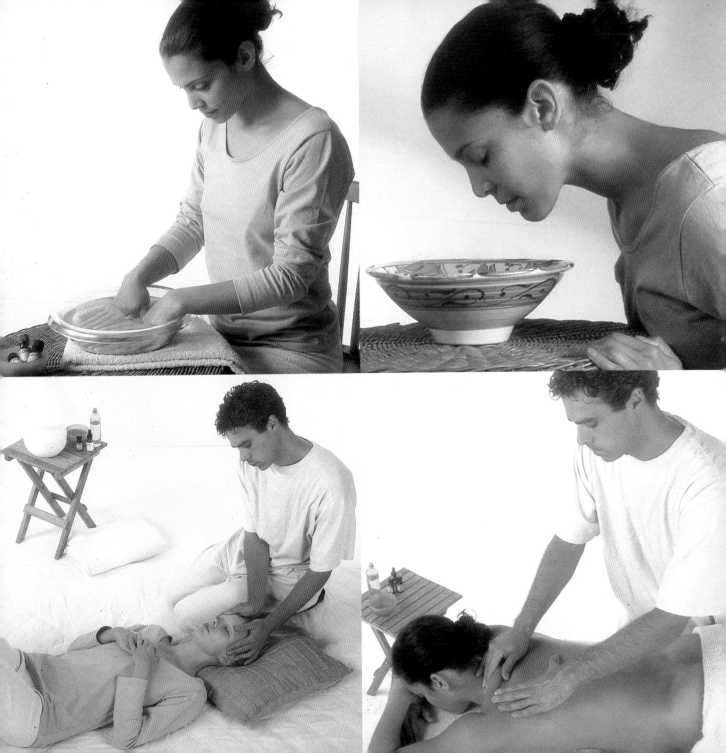

THE POWER OF SCENT: *the Art of Aromatherapy*

THE VALUE OF NATURAL PLANT OILS has been recognized for more than 5,000 years, for their healing, cleansing, preservative and mood-enhancing properties, as well as for the sheer pleasure of their fragrances. The art of aromatherapy harnesses these pure essences to work on the most powerful senses – smell and touch – to restore the harmony of body and mind. Use their beneficial properties to promote good health and emotional well-being, and to enhance every aspect of your life. These potent, volatile essences are nature's gift to mind and body.

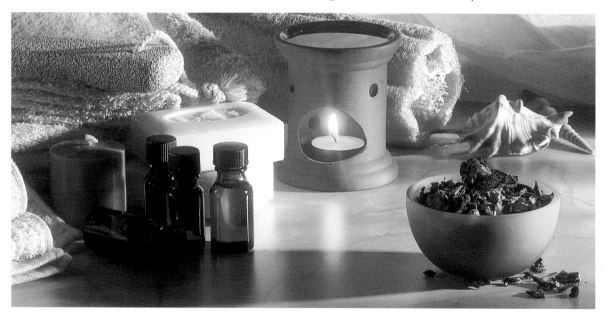

USING AND PREPARING OILS

AROMATIC ESSENTIAL OILS may be used in a number of ways to maintain and restore health, and to improve the quality of life with their scents. Essential oils are concentrated substances and as such they need to be diluted for safety and optimum effect. Treat them with care and respect – and allow them to treat you!

Essential oils are liable to deteriorate through the action of sunlight, so should be stored in a cool, dark place. They are sold in dark glass dropper bottles which protect the oils from the light and help with measuring. Only blend a small quantity of oils at a time to prevent the mixture deteriorating.

Many companies now sell essential oils; make sure that they are pure and of a high quality (you get what you pay for in general). If possible, try to smell a sample bottle of the oil you are buying in a shop – does it have a clean, non-synthetic odour with just one aromatic "note", or can you detect more than one scent? The latter may mean the oil is not so pure or fresh. Also beware of very cheap oils; what may seem to be a bargain may be of very little value for aromatherapy purposes and may even cause headaches or other reactions if used in excess.

For using essential oils at home, it can be helpful to have a little equipment. For vaporizing oils into the atmosphere, a burner is an easy option; simmering potpourri in a bowl with a candle underneath is another more unusual way to make a room fragrant, while a long-term scent, although fainter, can be achieved with a bowl of dry potpourri.

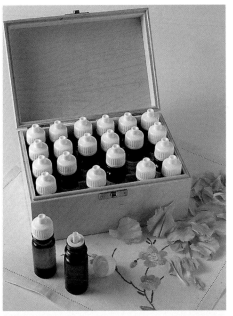

Keep essential oils in dark glass dropper bottles, out of the light to prevent deterioration by sunlight.

Right: Essential oils can be used in a burner or added to potpourri.

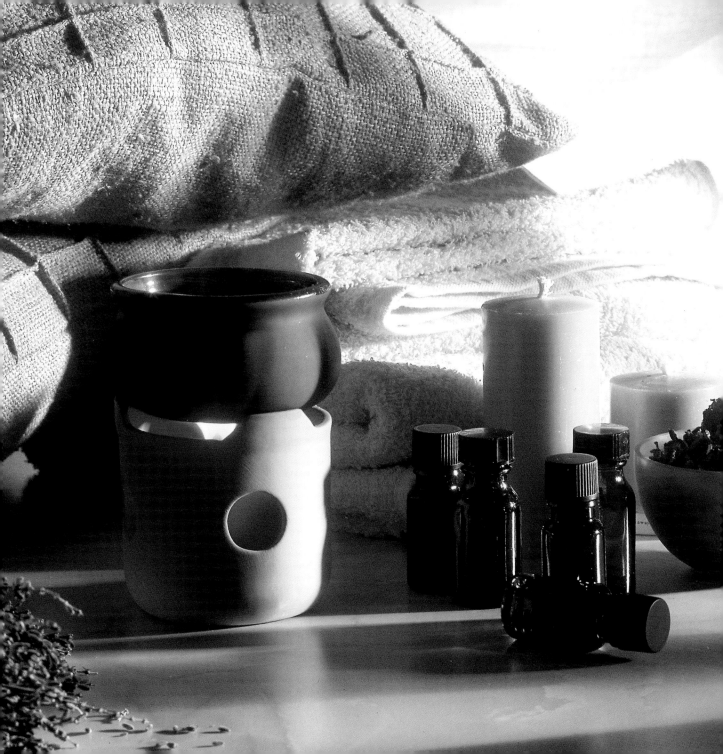

BATHS

Imagine soaking in a hot bath, enveloped in a delicious scent of exotic flowers, feeling all the day's tensions drop away . . . well, that can be a reality with aromatherapy. The oils seem to capture the essence of the plant, and can effortlessly transport you to pine-scented forests, refreshing orange groves or oriental spice markets.

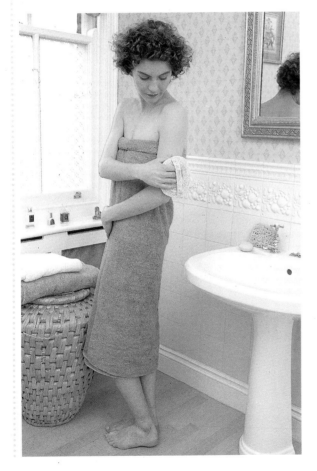

When using oils in the bath, pour in 5 drops just before you get in. The oils form a thin film on the surface of the water and this, aided by the warmth of the water, will be partly absorbed by your skin while you breathe in the scent, producing an immediate psychological and physiological effect.

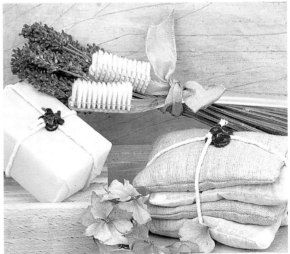

Left: Rubbing the body with a loofa increases the effectiveness of an aromatherapy bath. Above: Lavender has long been associated with bathing. Right: Essential oil in a burner will fragrance a room.

MORNING BATH

For a refreshing, uplifting bath in the mornings try a blend of 3 drops bergamot and 2 drops geranium essential oils.

EVENING BATH

To relax and unwind after a long day, make a blend of 3 drops lavender and 2 drops ylang ylang to add to your bath.

BATH FOR ACHING MUSCLES

For tired, tense muscles, soak in a bath to which you have added 3 drops marjoram and 2 drops chamomile essential oils.

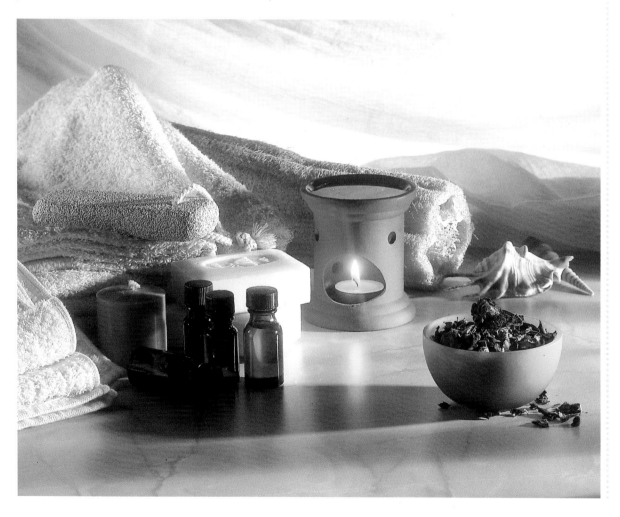

HAND AND FOOTBATHS

A quick way to use essential oils is to make a hand or footbath; two-thirds fill a large bowl with hot water and add 3–4 drops of oil. Circulation to our extremities is affected by tension and stress, among other things, and the warmth of the water itself helps the blood vessels to dilate. This can be very helpful in treating conditions such as tension headaches and migraines, when the blood vessels in the head are frequently engorged with blood. If you regularly suffer from these problems, try a foot or handbath at the first signs of a headache and see if you can drain away the excess stress.

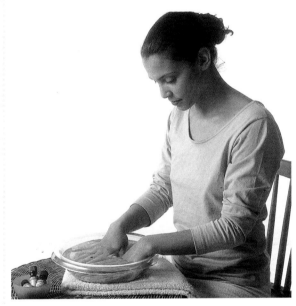

CIRCULATION
For poor circulation and tense, cold extremities, add 2 drops lavender and 2 drops marjoram oils.

ACHING MUSCLES: OVER-EXERTION
For tension and stiffness, perhaps from overuse, try a blend of 2 drops rosemary and 2 drops pine.

EXCESS HEAT: WHEN HOT AND BOTHERED
For hot, aching feet or hands, use a mixture of 2 drops peppermint and 2 drops lemon.

Left: Handbaths are a simple way of enjoying the benefits of essential oils. Below: Peppermint is cooling and counteracts tiredness. The essential oil is ideal for using in a refreshing footbath.

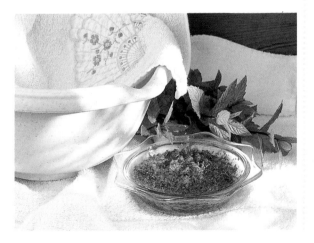

STEAM INHALATIONS

Colds and sinus problems may cause congestion, but we can also feel blocked up and unable to breathe freely through tension. Using a steam inhalation warms and moistens the membranes, and the use of essential oils helps to open and relax the airways. Just boil a kettle, pour the water into a bowl, add the oils and inhale deeply.

NASAL CONGESTION

For a stuffed-up feeling, maybe combined with tiredness, try using 3 drops eucalyptus and 2 drops peppermint in a bowl of steaming water.

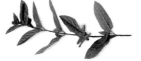

TIGHT, TENSE CHEST

For tension causing poor breathing, relax the airways with 4 drops lavender and 3 drops frankincense.

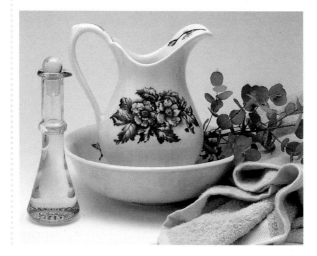

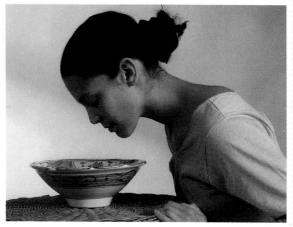

Above: For respiratory complaints in particular, steam inhalations are very helpful. Use a total of 10 drops for a strong medicinal effect, in cases of colds and chestiness, or just 5 drops for a gentler relaxing effect on the airways. Left: Eucalyptus is particularly effective at clearing the chest and nose.

CAUTION:
If you have high blood pressure or asthma seek medical advice before using steam, and in any case do not overdo an inhalation.

SCENTED ROOMS

Aromatherapy has many applications in the home or office including the creation
of an aromatic environment which has wide-ranging beneficial effects.

POTPOURRI

It is possible to scent a room by making a simmering
potpourri. Place a mixture of scented flowers and
leaves (without any fixatives or additives) in a bowl of
water and heat gently from below – a candle may well
be sufficient. Unlike dry potpourri, the simmering
variety does not last for long but gives off a much
stronger aroma at the time. Try making your own
blends, using your nose to achieve the aroma you
desire; add about 1 cupful of dried material to
1.2 litres (2 pints) of water.

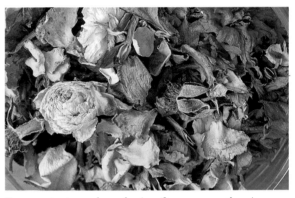

Potpourri gives a long-lasting fragrance to the air.

For a sleep-enhancing simmering potpourri
blend try using ½ cup lime flowers, ¼ cup
chamomile flowers, 1 tbsp sweet marjoram and 1 tbsp
lavender flowers. For a more refreshing, uplifting
blend try mixing together ½ cup lemon verbena
leaves, ¼ cup jasmine flowers, 2 tbsp lemon peel and
1 tsp coriander seeds.

ESSENTIAL OIL BURNERS

Most oils lend themselves to use in a burner. The
basic principle is very simple: a small dish to hold a
few drops of essential oil, with some type of gentle
heat underneath, often in the form of a candle. The
heat needs to be fairly low, in order to allow slow
evaporation of the oil and a longer-lasting scent.

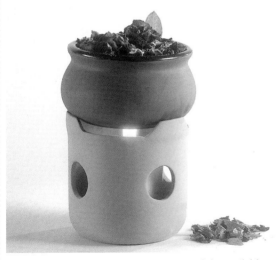

Special potpourri burners are now widely available.

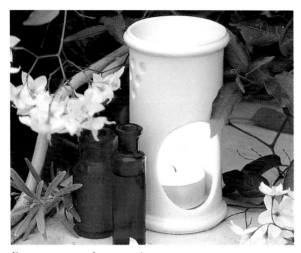

Burners can make attractive room ornaments.

If you want to fumigate a room, then try adding 3–4 drops of oils such as pine, eucalyptus or juniper to a burner. To help you keep alert, then a couple of drops of peppermint or rosemary may be appropriate, while 2–3 drops of ylang ylang or lavender will help you to wind down at the end of the day.

BOWL OF HOT WATER

Adding a couple of drops of an essential oil to a bowl of hot water can be a pleasant way to give fragrance to a room or office, especially if the atmosphere is dry as a result of central heating. Choose an attractive bowl and place it out of reach of children. Use an oil that you really like, as its scent will linger for some time.

For mornings, one of the fresh aromas such as bergamot, mandarin or lemon would be uplifting. Later in the day you may wish to use a floral essence, such as rose or jasmine, which have calming effects.

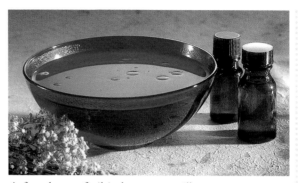

A few drops of oil in hot water will scent a room.

OTHER SCENTED PRODUCTS

Essential oils are quite often included in items such as scented candles, incense sticks or cones, and other aromatic products. It is important to check that natural essential oils have been used to scent these products before you buy them; synthetic perfumes may have a similar scent but they will not have the beneficial therapeutic properties of natural plant extracts.

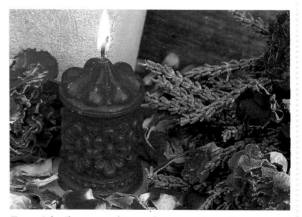

Essential oils are used to make scented candles.

COMPRESSES

Hot or cold compresses are excellent ways to use oils for problems such as sprains and muscular aches. To make a cold compress, pour cold water over some ice in a bowl, add essential oils and soak a pad in the water before placing over the affected area and binding firmly in place. For a hot compress, have the water as hot as you can comfortably bear and pour into a bowl, add oils and use as above. Use 3–4 drops of essential oils in an average sized cereal bowl.

Cold compresses are suitable for use on acute injuries such as a strain or sprain, with swelling or bruising. For older injuries, with no swelling or inflammation, for chronic muscle aches such as backache and menstrual pain, and for arthritic or rheumatic pain, a hot compress may be more useful.

The ideal essential oil for a cold compress is lavender, and this can be very useful in many first aid situations. Use 4 drops to a bowl of iced water. Keep the pad on firmly for at least 20 minutes, preferably with the affected limb raised if there is any swelling.

For muscular aches and pains, try using 2 drops of both rosemary and marjoram in a bowl of hot water. Apply the compress for 30 minutes.

CAUTION:
For any major injury always seek medical advice or treatment.

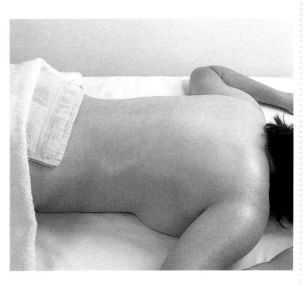

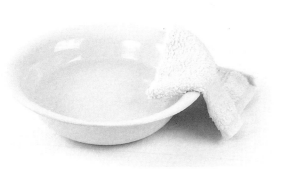

Left: Aromatherapy oils can be added to warm water to make a soothing compress. Above: Compresses can stimulate circulation and reduce inflammation.

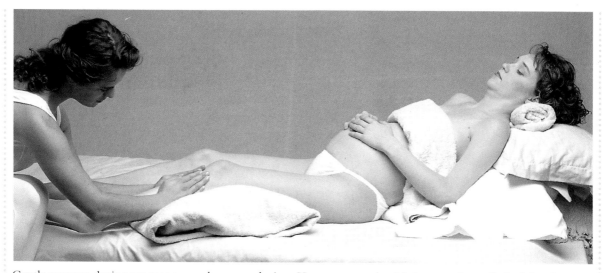

Gentle massage during pregnancy can be very relaxing. However, you should always seek medical advice first.

CAUTION:

Essential oils are wonderful natural remedies for a variety of problems, and their aromatic effects can enhance mood, release tensions and reduce stress. But they are highly concentrated substances and must be used with caution. Follow the advice given below and if in any doubt seek a medical opinion before using them.

• Never take essential oils internally, unless professionally prescribed.

• Always use essential oils diluted – normally 1 per cent for massage; just 5 drops in a bath or for a steam inhalation.

• Do not use the same oils for too long, follow the "1–2 rule"; use one or two oils together, for not more than one or two weeks at any one time.

• Do not use oils in pregnancy, without getting professional advice; some oils, such as basil, clary sage, juniper, marjoram and sage, are contra-indicated at this time.

• For anyone who has any skin problems, dilute the oils even more and if any skin irritation occurs stop using them immediately. A few essential oils, such as bergamot, make the skin more sensitive to sunlight, so should be used with caution in hot, sunny weather.

• Be extra careful with anyone who has asthma or epilepsy, and if anyone experiences a reaction, then stop using the oil.

THE OILS

ESSENTIAL OILS MAY BE EXTRACTED from exotic plants such as sandalwood or ylang ylang, or from more common plants like lavender and chamomile, but each one has its own characteristics and properties. Try to get used to a few oils at first, understand their effects, and enjoy their fragrance!

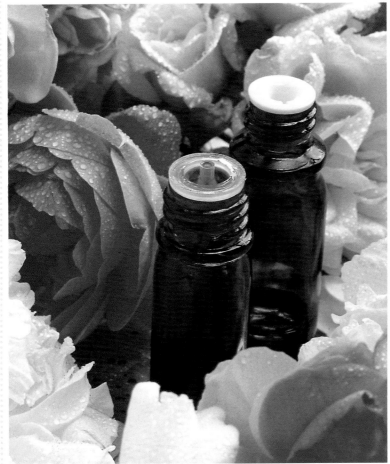

Left: Essential oils are concentrated substances; while the skin of citrus fruits such as lemon or orange may yield a fair amount of oil, flowers such as roses only contain tiny amounts of the precious essence – about 5,000 roses may be needed to obtain 5 ml (1 tsp) of pure essential oil. This concentration emphasizes the importance of only using drop doses of the oils, in a suitable dilution, as a little goes a long way.

Right: Oils are extracted from many different parts of plants. Each contains powerful healing properties, to be enjoyed but also respected. Nature provides an abundance of therapeutic compounds to help us regain health and vitality.

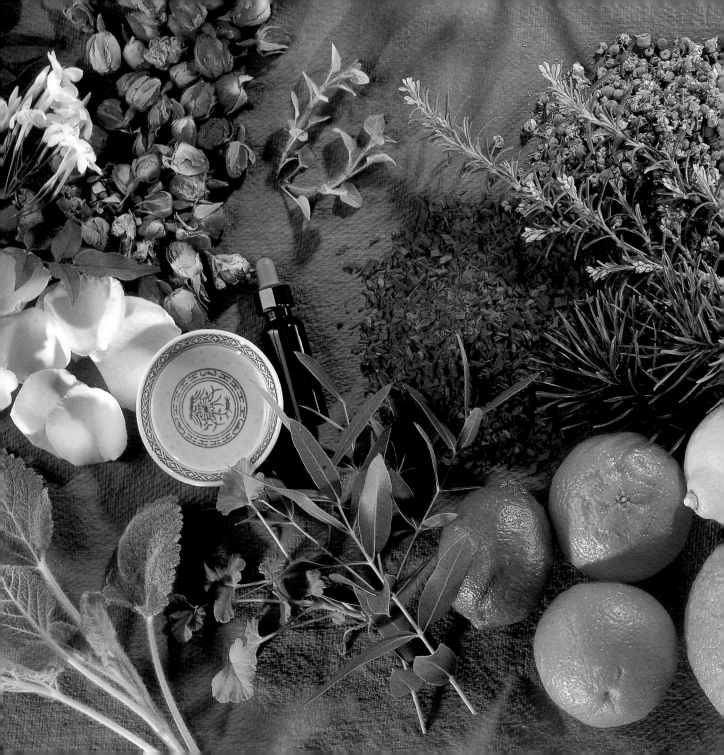

SANDALWOOD (*SANTALUM ALBUM*)
Probably the oldest perfume in history,
known to have been used for over 4,000
years. Sandalwood has a heavy scent, and
often appeals to men as much as to
women. It has a relaxing, antidepressant
effect on the nervous system, and where
depression causes sexual problems,
sandalwood can be a genuine aphrodisiac.

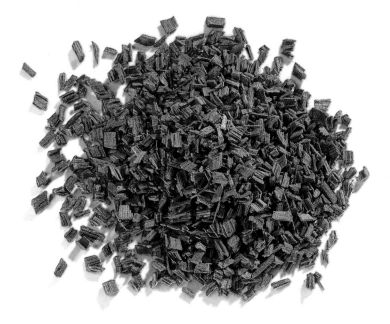

CHAMOMILE (*MATRICARIA RECUTITA*
[German] or *CHAMAEMELUM NOBILE*
[Roman])
Roman and German chamomile are both used to
obtain essential oils with very similar properties.
Chamomile is relaxing and antispasmodic,
helping to relieve tension headaches, nervous
digestive problems or insomnia, for instance.

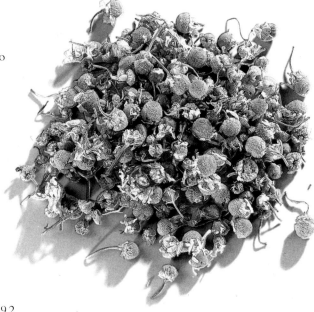

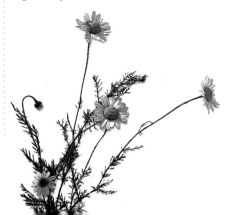

BENZOIN (*STYRAX BENZOIN*)

This Asiatic tree produces a gum which is usually dissolved in a solvent to produce the "oil". It has a wonderful fragrance of vanilla, and is widely used in inhalation mixtures. It relaxes the airways and can be used whenever tension leads to a tight chest or restricted breathing.

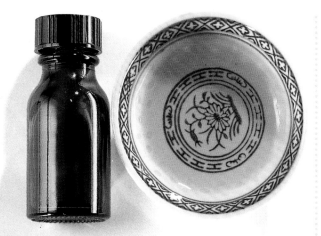

GERANIUM (*PELARGONIUM GRAVEOLENS*)

The rose-scented geranium has very useful properties, not least being its ability to bring a blend together, to make a more harmonious scent. Geranium has a refreshing, antidepressant quality, good for nervous tension and exhaustion.

YLANG YLANG (*CANANGA ODORATA* VAR. *GENUINA*)

This tropical tree, native to Indonesia, produces an intensely sweet essential oil that has a sedative yet antidepressant action. It is good for many symptoms of excessive tension such as insomnia, panic attacks, anxiety and depression. It also has a good reputation as an aphrodisiac, through its ability to reduce stress levels.

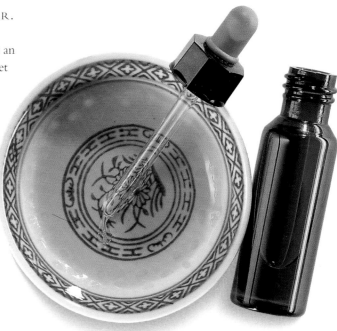

PEPPERMINT (*MENTHA PIPERITA*)

This oil is another classic ingredient in inhalations for relieving catarrh, although commercially menthol (a major part of the oil) may be used. Peppermint's analgesic and antispasmodic effects make it very useful for rubbing on to the temples to ease tension headaches; ideally dilute a drop in a little base cream or oil before applying.

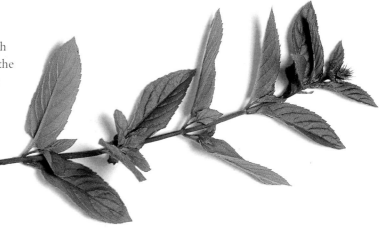

JASMINE (*JASMINUM OFFICINALE*)
One of the most wonderful aromas, jasmine has
a relaxing, euphoric effect, and can greatly lift
the mood when there is debility, depression and
listlessness. Use in the bath or in massage oils,
or use jasmine flower water for oily skin.

EUCALYPTUS (*EUCALYPTUS GLOBULUS*)
One of the finest oils for respiratory complaints, found
in most commercial inhalants. Well diluted (never use
more than 1 per cent) in a base vegetable oil, it can
be applied to the forehead to help relieve a hot,
tense headache linked with tiredness.

LAVENDER (*LAVANDULA ANGUSTIFOLIA*)

One of the most well-known scents, lavender has been used for centuries to refresh and add fragrance to the home, and as a remedy for stress-related ailments. It is especially helpful for tension headaches, or for nervous digestive upsets; use in a massage oil or in the bath for a deeply relaxing and calming experience.

The finest oil is produced from the true lavender (*Lavandula angustifolia*), and is one of the safest and most versatile of all oils. Its uses range from first-aid treatment of burns, to skin care products, oils for muscular aches and pains, smelling salts for shock, and a host of stress-reducing applications.

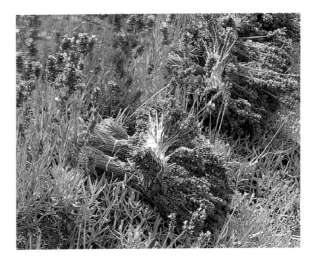

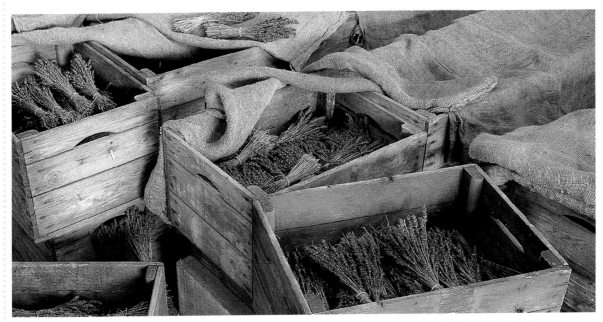

Lavender used to be grown extensively in England, but today France and Spain are the principal producers.

ROSEMARY (*ROSMARINUS OFFICINALIS*)
With a very penetrating, stimulating aroma, rosemary
has been used for centuries to help to relieve nervous
exhaustion, tension headaches and migraines. It
improves circulation to the brain, and is an excellent
oil for mental fatigue and debility.

MARJORAM (*ORIGANUM MARJORANA*)
Marjoram has a calming and warming effect, and
is good for both cold, tight muscles and for
cold, tense people who might suffer from
headaches, migraines and insomnia. Use in
massage blends for rubbing into tired and
aching muscles, or in the bath, especially
in the evening to help to obtain a good
night's sleep.

PINE (*PINUS SYLVESTRIS*)
There are a few species of pine that produce oils,
notably the American long-leaf pine which is a
commercial source of oil of turpentine. However,
the pine oil used in aromatherapy generally
comes from the Scots pine. It helps to clear
the air passages when used as an inhalation,
and is also good for relieving fatigue. Tired,
aching muscles can be eased with massage
using diluted pine oil.

CLARY SAGE (*SALVIA SCLAREA*)
This oil gives a definite euphoric uplift to the brain;
do not use too much, however, as you can be left
feeling very spacey! Like ylang ylang and jasmine,
its antidepressant and relaxing qualities have
contributed to its reputation as an
aphrodisiac.

ROSE *(ROSA X DAMASCENA, CENTIFOLIA)*

Rose is probably the most famous of all oils, prized since the beginning of time both as a marvellous fragrance and as a valuable remedy for many ailments. There is probably more symbolism attached to roses than any other flower, and their scent can evoke a general sense of pleasure and happiness.

Several kinds of roses have been used to extract the oil, notably the damask rose and the cabbage rose. Each one is slightly different, but the overall actions are sedating, calming and anti-inflammatory. Not surprisingly, rose oil has a wide reputation as an aphrodisiac, and where anxiety is a factor, it may be very beneficial. Use in the bath for a sensual, unwinding experience, or add to a base massage oil to soothe muscular and nervous tension.

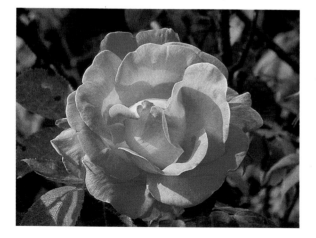

Rose (*Rosa* species)

CITRUS OILS

Many citrus fruits yield essential oils, and they tend to have similar properties. In general they are refreshing, stimulating oils, good for the morning bath, leaving you feeling cleansed and alive.

BERGAMOT (*CITRUS BERGAMIA*)

The peel of the ripe fruit yields an oil that is mild and gentle. It is the most effective antidepressant oil of all, best used at the start of the day. Its leaves give the distinctive aroma and flavour to Earl Grey tea. The oil can be used on a burner for generally lifting the atmosphere. Do not use on the skin in bright sunlight, as it increases photosensitivity.

BITTER ORANGE (*CITRUS AURANTIUM* VAR. *AMARA*)

The bitter, or Seville, orange is the source of not one but three different oils, from the fruit, the blossom (also called neroli) and the leaf (also called petitgrain). These have overlapping effects; neroli is especially good as a tonic and mood lifter, raising the spirits and maybe the libido.

LEMON (*CITRUS LIMON*)

Possibly the most cleansing and antiseptic of the citrus oils, useful for boosting the immune system and in skin care. It can also refresh and clarify thoughts.

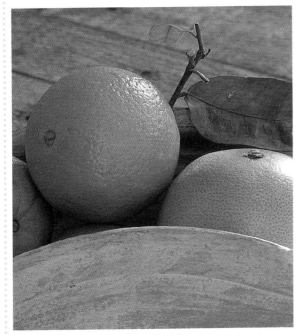

Citrus oils are great tonics, having a fresh, stimulating aroma to lift the mood and spirits.

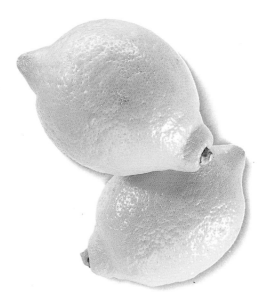

MANDARIN (*CITRUS RETICULATA*)

Refreshing and cleansing, this sweetly scented oil is especially good for skin problems such as acne. It also helps digestion, soothing heartburn and nausea.

GRAPEFRUIT (*CITRUS X PARADISI*)

Oil of grapefruit is very helpful in the digestion of fatty foods and helps to combat cellulite and congested pores. It has an uplifting effect and will soothe headaches and nervous exhaustion.

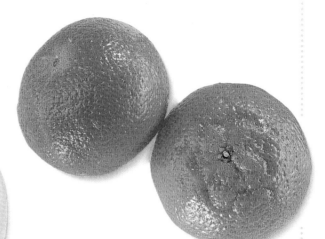

LIMES (*CITRUS AURANTIFOLIA*)

Oil of lime is good for stimulating a sluggish system and may be used when a tonic is needed, in massage or in the bath.

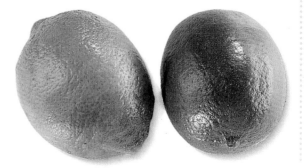

THERAPEUTIC RECIPES

ONE OF THE DELIGHTS of aromatherapy is the blending together of oils for an enhanced therapeutic effect, with a new fragrance to soothe the senses at the same time. On the following pages you will find ideas for using combinations of oils; these have been created for their healing properties, but they also combine well in aroma. The sense of smell is very individual, so if you do not like a particular combination, try making your own blends, bearing in mind the actions of the oils and the dilution rates described earlier.

Try to ensure you buy good quality essential oils, with a pure scent that comes from the natural, unadulterated extract. Let your nose

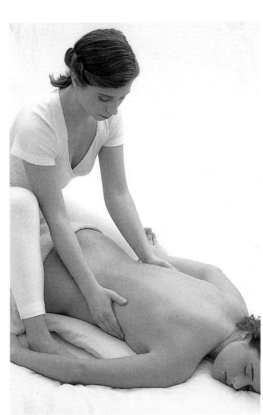

Taking time to relax and unwind with an aromatherapy massage is a wonderful and natural way to ease the body of stored tensions.

tell you of the quality and if a blend is harmonious, but above all if you enjoy the aroma.

For each of the blends suggested in this section, the number of drops of oils given should be diluted for massage purposes in 20 ml (4 tsp) of a base vegetable oil such as sweet almond oil. For a steam inhalation, use the number of drops given in a large bowl holding about 1 litre (1¾ pints) of hot water, and for a compress add the specified number of oil drops to a bowl holding 250 ml (8 fl oz) of hot water.

Right: Using essential oils in your daily routine is not only pleasurable but is also a means of improving your health and vitality.

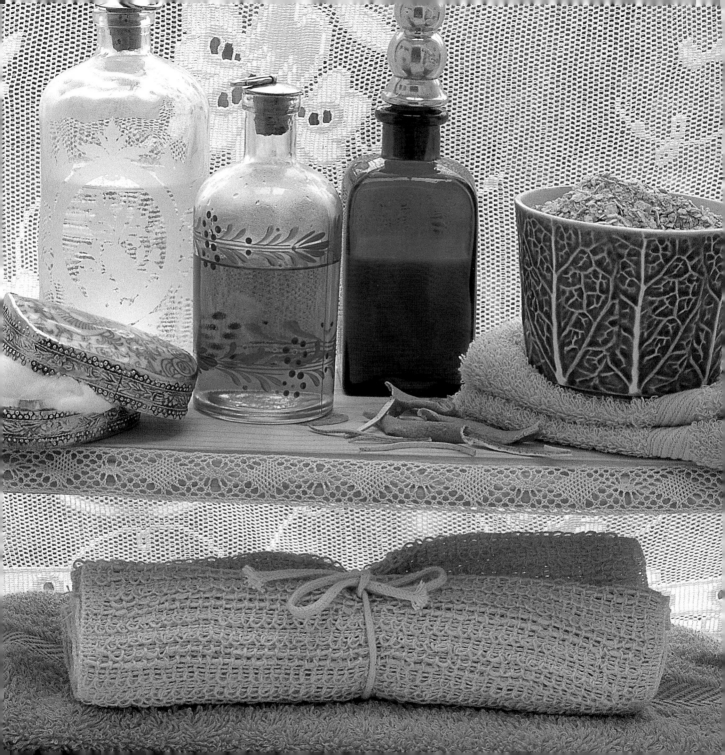

ANXIETY CALMERS

When people are described as being "uptight", that is often exactly what they are: tense muscles in the face and neck are a sure sign of anxiety. Release that tension with a face massage, using gentle, soothing strokes on the temples and forehead especially. This is very good as an evening treat, calming away the day's cares and worries.

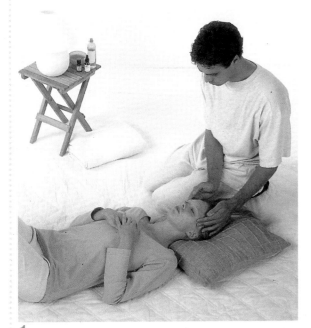

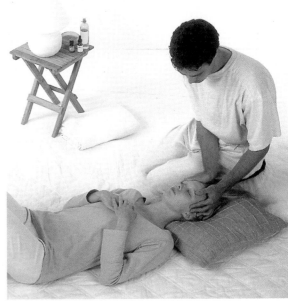

1 Ideally have the person lying down with the head in your lap or on a cushion. With your fingertips, gently smooth the essential oil blend into the face and head to aid relaxation.

Use just a little oil, as most people do not like a greasy feeling on the face. Make up a blend of 4 drops lavender and 2 drops ylang ylang in a light oil such as sweet almond, grapeseed or coconut.

2 Using your thumbs one after the other, stroke tension away from the centre of the forehead.

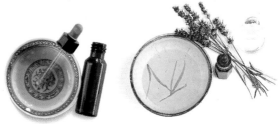

BACKACHE SOOTHERS

So often people carry around their tensions in the form of a stiff, aching or knotted back. Symptoms can range from tight shoulders to lower backache, and the best way of using the essential oils is in massage of the taut muscles. Use long, sweeping strokes and a deeper kneading action to loosen areas of spasm, and let the aromatic oils work their magic at the same time.

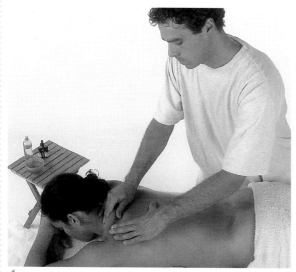

1 Knead the shoulders to ease stiff muscles.

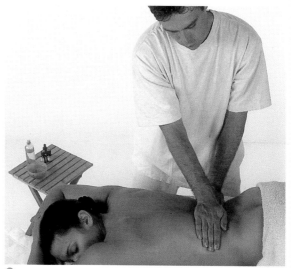

2 Apply steady, sweeping movements with the hands.

◀ 3 Stroke firmly down the back with both hands.

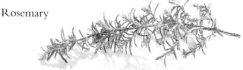
Rosemary

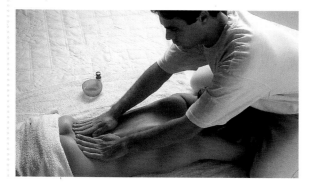

Two essential oil blends that will help to work on the deeper tensions and knotted muscles are 3 drops pine and 3 drops rosemary, or 4 drops lavender and 3 drops marjoram mixed with the base oil.

UPLIFTING OILS

There are unfortunately times in all our lives when we get depressed to some extent, whether due to a specific event or from chronic tiredness. As part of a programme of recuperation and restoring vitality, aromatherapy can be very effective in lifting the mood and overall energy.

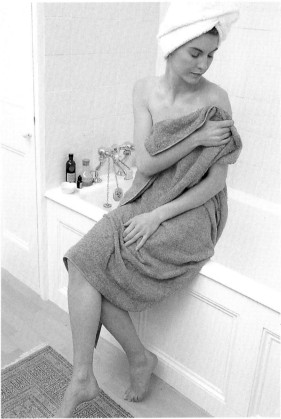

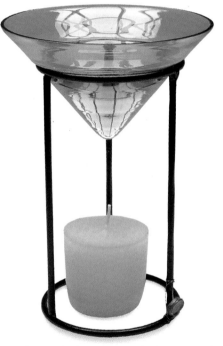

A gentler effect, which can pervade the atmosphere all day long, is to use bergamot or neroli oils in an essential oil burner – probably just one drop of each oil at a time, repeating as needed.

For a strong, but relatively short-lived effect, try 4 drops bergamot and 2 drops neroli in the bath, ideally in the morning. After the bath, gently pat the skin with a soft towel. Do not rub vigorously.

SKIN TONICS

When we become stressed, the small muscles close to the skin tend to contract. This can leave our skin under-nourished with blood, and over time our complexion and skin tone suffer. Apart from dealing with the underlying worries, the skin itself can also be helped with essential oils. Tense skin is frequently drier than normal, and probably the best way to use the oils is to mix them into your favourite skin cream. Obviously this is best if the cream is originally unperfumed.

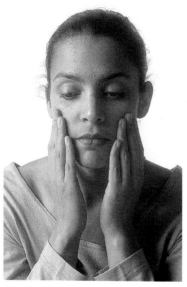

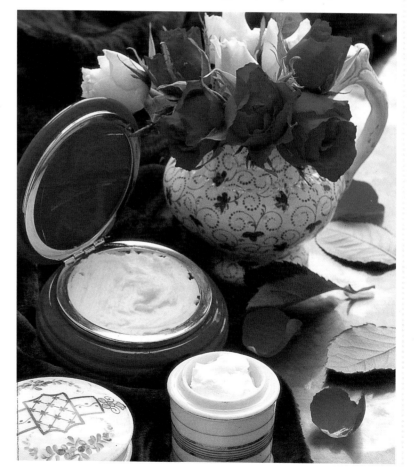

Above: To a 25 g (1oz) pot of skin cream, add either 3 drops rose and 3 drops sandalwood, or 4 drops neroli and 2 drops rose and apply to the skin.

Right: As with all essential oil blends, it is best if you only mix up small amounts of cream and oil at a time.

HEADACHE EASERS

Tension headaches are a common feature in many people's lives, and may come from long hours at the computer or even longer hours with small children! Whatever the cause, gentle massage of the temples and forehead at the earliest moment can help to stop headaches from getting a tight grip. Another option is a warm compress.

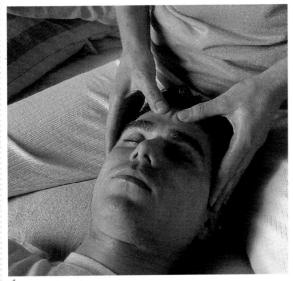

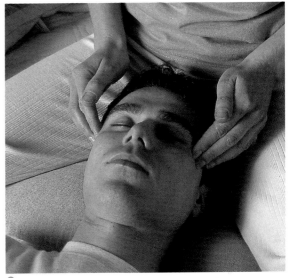

1 Ease tension headaches by massaging oils into the forehead. With your thumbs, use steady but gentle pressure to stroke the forehead.

2 Gently massage the temples with the fingers to release tension and stress.

• If the head feels hot, try using an oil with 4 drops peppermint.
• If warmth feels as though it is helpful, use 6 drops lavender.
• Another option for either type of headache is 4 drops chamomile.

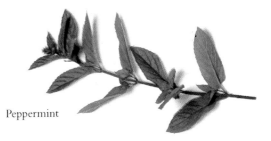

Peppermint

HIGH BLOOD PRESSURE RELIEVER

It should be emphasized that anyone with very high blood pressure should first seek medical (or professional) treatment. In milder cases, related to anxiety and tension, you can help to get temporary relief by using essential oils. A very good way to do so is in a footbath, the warmth from the water helping to bring blood to the feet and reduce the blood pressure.

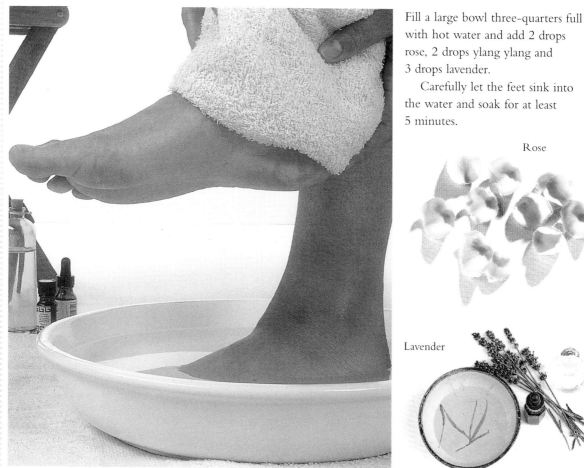

Fill a large bowl three-quarters full with hot water and add 2 drops rose, 2 drops ylang ylang and 3 drops lavender.

Carefully let the feet sink into the water and soak for at least 5 minutes.

Rose

Lavender

CELLULITE REDUCERS

Cellulite, which collects mostly on the hips, buttocks and upper arms, is not specifically related to body weight and affects people of all sizes, especially women. It is caused by toxic deposits in the fatty tissues and is detectable by the bumpy "orange peel" look of the skin in these problem areas.

A build-up of cellulite usually results from a sluggish circulation and poor elimination of toxins from the body. To improve the condition you need to use a combination of approaches. Review your diet and cut down on your intake of toxins such as refined carbohydrates, caffeine and alcohol. Increase the amount of fresh vegetables and water. Fennel tea is a natural diuretic which will aid the elimination of toxins. Regular exercise is also important, as it helps the lymphatic system rid the body of waste products.

Massage with the recommended essential oils should become part of your daily routine for 6–8 weeks to help achieve a smooth and healthy skin. Mechanical massage instruments are helpful for this. You can try a quick self-massage several times a day, such as when dressing or after taking a bath or shower. Squeeze and knead the thighs and buttocks, and follow up with percussion movements.

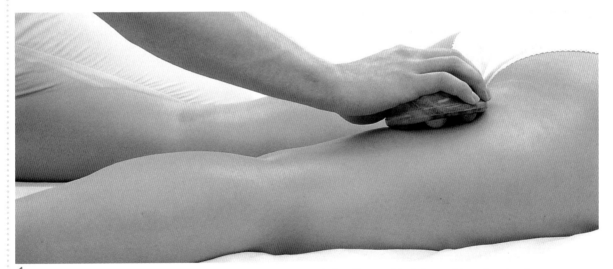

1 Hand-held massage instruments such as this wooden six-ball roller are ideal for making the circular pressure motions that help to smooth out cellulite spots on the thighs.

The following blend will stimulate circulation, detoxify the system and help prevent water retention: 3 drops lemon, 2 drops geranium, 2 drops fennel and 1 drop black pepper.

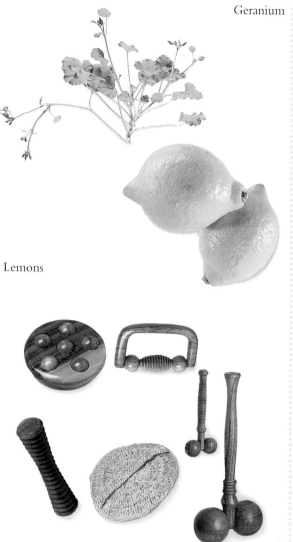

Geranium

Lemons

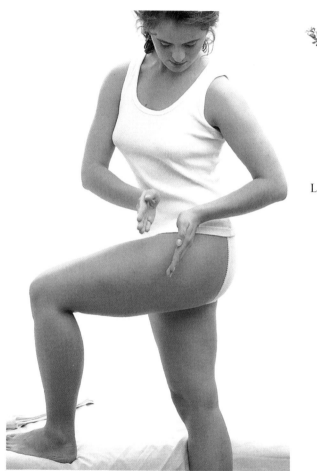

2 Hack, cup and pummel the thighs briskly to tone the area and revitalize the blood circulation.

Above: Massage tools are particularly useful for aiding self-massage.

NIGHT-TIME SOOTHERS

Worries can go round and round inside our heads, usually just as we are trying to get to sleep. The resulting disturbed and restless night leaves us more prone to stress and anxiety, and a vicious cycle can be created. Help break this cycle with a pleasantly hot and relaxing evening bath. Many oils can be useful – just having a fragrance that you enjoy will help you to unwind after a long day.

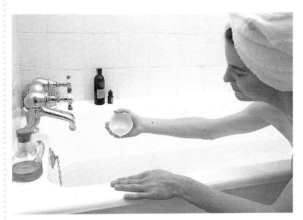

Above: Add oils to an evening bath to aid relaxation and sleep. A couple of relaxing blends, without over-sedating, are 4 drops rose and 3 drops sandalwood or 5 drops lavender and 3 drops ylang ylang.

Right: Incorporate aromatherapy preparations into your daily bathing routine.

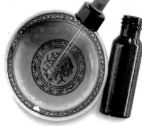

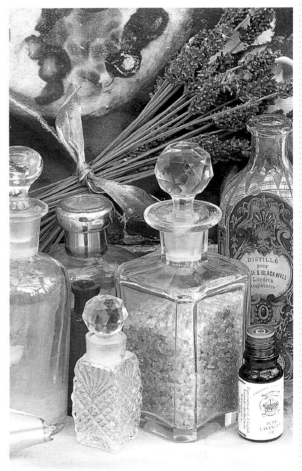

INVIGORATING OILS

Chronic tension all too often leads to a feeling of exhaustion, when we just run out of steam. At these times we need a boost, and many oils have a tonic effect, restoring vitality without over-stimulating. As a group, the citrus oils are good for this purpose, ranging from the more soothing mandarin to the very refreshing lemon oil.

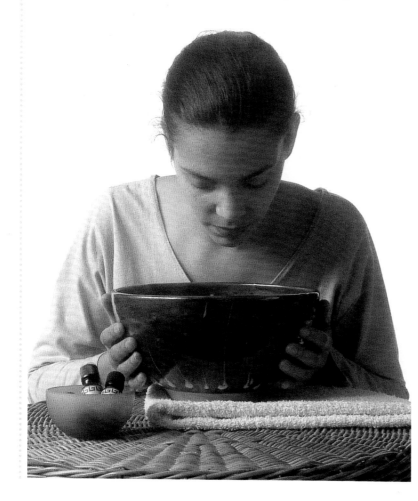

Have a warm, but not too hot bath, with 4 drops mandarin and 2 drops orange or 4 drops neroli and 2 drops lemon. Alternatively, just add a couple of drops of any of these oils to a bowl of steaming water and gently inhale to help to clear away the tiredness and lift your spirits.

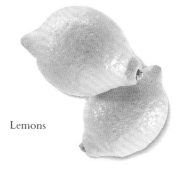

Lemons

Left: Steam inhalation is a valuable and simple way to receive the benefits of essential oils when time or circumstance prevent massage or a bath.

MENSTRUAL PAIN RELIEVERS

Painful periods can be due to a number of reasons, but tension will certainly add to muscle spasm and cramping pains. If there is no organic or structural cause of the discomfort, try using essential oils, either as a hot compress over the lower abdomen or in the bath. Some oils have a reputation for improving the menstrual cycle in other ways; seek advice from a professional aromatherapist for longer-term treatments.

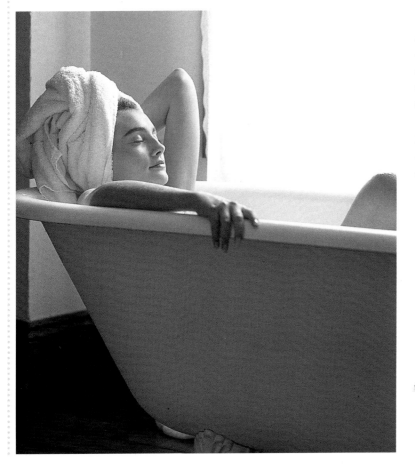

For a compress, use 1 drop of rose, geranium and clary sage oils. Alternatively, a fairly hot bath with 3 drops rose, 3 drops geranium and 2 drops clary sage will quickly relax cramped muscles.

Left: A long bath with a few drops of oil will help you to relax and to soothe away any discomfort.

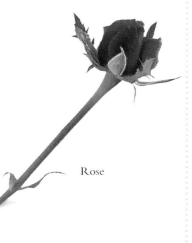

Rose

PRE-MENSTRUAL TENSION SOOTHERS

For many women the days leading up to a period can be fraught with mood swings, irritability and other symptoms. Professional treatment may be needed for full assistance; however, try this blend of oils if before each period you feel very tense and critical of those around you, or just want to devour a box of chocolates!

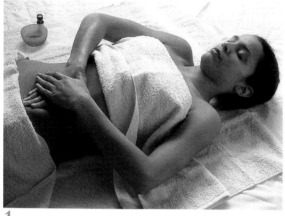

1 Slowly and firmly massage the abdomen with your hands.

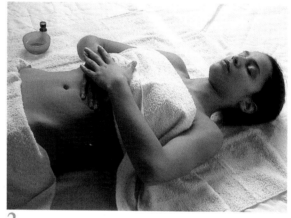

2 Move your hands in a clockwise direction; try to remain relaxed the whole time.

Either add 3 drops rose, 3 drops jasmine and 2 drops clary sage to a bath and lie back allowing the tension to soak away, or use this mixture in a massage oil and rub gently into the abdomen for a relaxing, soothing effect.

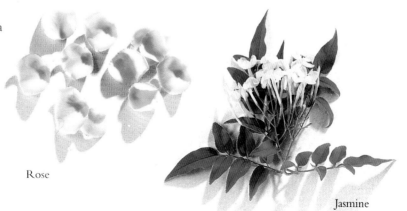

Rose

Jasmine

MIGRAINE EASERS

One of the most complex of health problems, migraines are nature's way of shutting us down when life has been too demanding. The triggers that spark off a migraine attack are highly individual and professional treatment is really needed to try to understand the causes for each person. Many migraine sufferers have a heightened sense of smell at the onset of the attack and may find any aroma intolerable, so use oils sparingly and carefully.

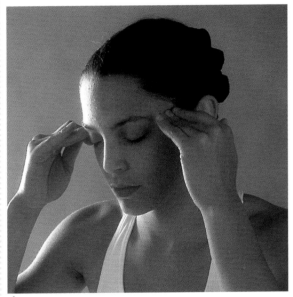

1 For self-help, gently massage the temples with small circling movements.

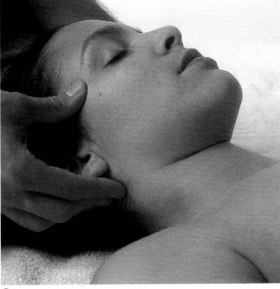

2 A gentle head massage from a partner can be even more beneficial.

At the earliest stage of a migraine, try using a blend of 2 drops rosemary, 1 drop marjoram and 1 drop clary sage, diluted in a massage oil and very gently massaged into the temples and forehead. Alternatively, use a drop of each oil in a bowl of warm water and apply a compress to the forehead.

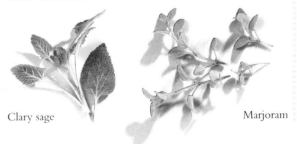

Clary sage

Marjoram

MILD SHOCK SOOTHERS

You bump your head, trip over the cat, fall down the stairs, get the gas bill . . . we all have times when we get rather shaken up and suffer from mild shock. We may feel a little dizzy or faint, and need to sit down. At these times, essential oils can be a useful first-aid help, bringing us back to our senses.

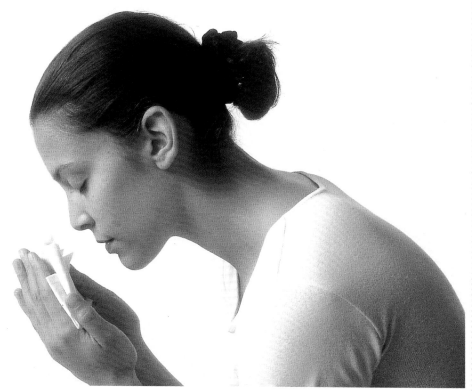

The quickest and simplest way to benefit from aromatherapy in instances of mild shock is to put an open bottle of either lavender or clary sage oil under the person's nose and let them sniff the aroma directly. Otherwise, put a couple of oil drops on a tissue, hold under the nose and inhale.

CAUTION:
Remember, never try to treat a case of severe shock at home. Seek medical advice immediately.

MUSCULAR ACHE RELIEVERS

When you are under stress for any length of time, your body stays permanently tense. This can make any or all of your muscles ache and feel tired or heavy. To relieve these symptoms, and also to begin to release the underlying tension, use essential oils in a massage blend. As the massage movements work on the aching muscles, the oils are being absorbed and get to work on inner tension too.

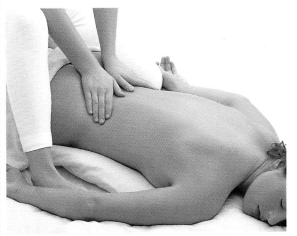

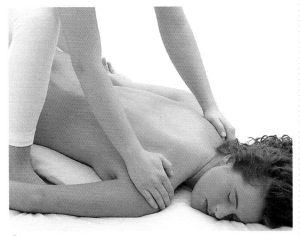

1 Rest your hands on the lower back either side of the spine. Lean your weight into your hands and stroke firmly up the back towards the head. Mould your hands to the body as they glide along.

2 As your hands reach the top of the back, fan them out towards the shoulders in a flowing motion.

Marjoram

Use a blend of 3 drops pine, 3 drops marjoram and 2 drops juniper for a variety of soothing massage strokes.

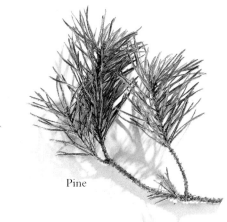

Pine

118

REVITALIZING OILS

In today's high pressure world, trying to juggle with too many demands leads nearly all of us to reach a state of "brain fag" at some point, when mental fatigue and exhaustion grind us to a halt. Rather than reach for the coffee, or worse still alcohol, which may seem to relax but actually depresses the central nervous system, try using these revitalizing oils to give you an instant pick-me-up and make you feel more alert.

Below: You can use 1–2 drops of rosemary or peppermint oil in a burner. Alternatively, add 3 drops rosemary and 2 drops peppermint to a bowl of steaming water, or use 4 drops of either oils on their own. Allow the oils to evaporate into the room and breathe freely.

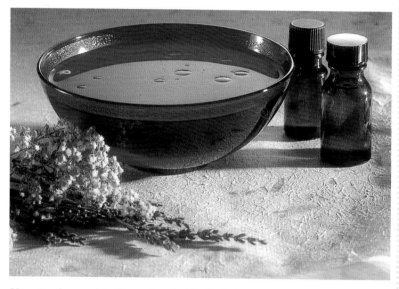

Vaporized essential oils are invaluable for balancing the emotions.

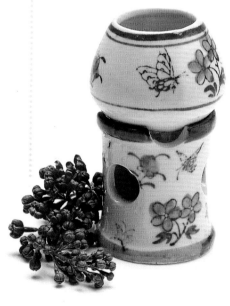

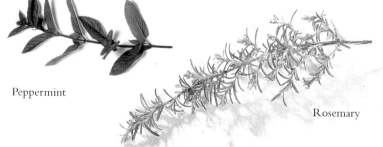

Peppermint

Rosemary

STRESS REDUCERS

Stress, or rather our inability to cope with an excess amount of it, is one of the biggest health problems today. Lifestyles seem to include so many demands that it is not surprising that most of us feel stressed at times, sometimes constantly. We all react to excessive stress in different ways, with tension, anxiety, depression or exhaustion, but we can all benefit from the wonderfully balancing and stress-busting effects of aromatic oils.

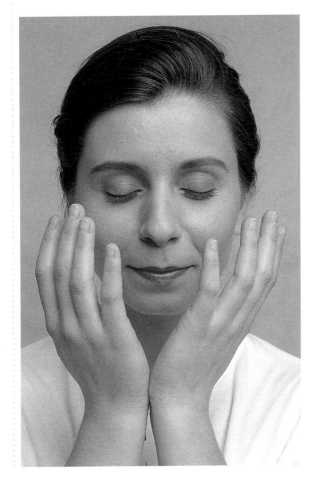

Our bodies are geared to cope with a stressful situation by producing various hormones that trigger off a series of physiological actions in the body; these are known collectively as the "fight or flight" syndrome, and serve to place the body in a state of alert in a potentially dangerous situation. Extra blood is shunted to the muscles, and the heart rate speeds up while the digestion slows down. These responses are appropriate when we are faced with a physical threat, but can nowadays be triggered by quite different kinds of stress and end up placing a strain on our bodies without fulfilling any useful need.

.In order to help reduce the impact of stress on the whole system, it is necessary to find ways both to avoid getting over-stressed in the first instance and to let go of the changes that occur internally under stress. Aromatherapy can help in each case, the oils helping to keep you calm under pressure and releasing inner tensions following stress, especially in massage.

To prevent undue stress, try simply inhaling one of your favourite oils at regular intervals, or put a couple of drops in a burner in your room or office, to help keep you feeling more relaxed and calm.

Left: It should not take you long to discover which essential oils work best for you as an individual.

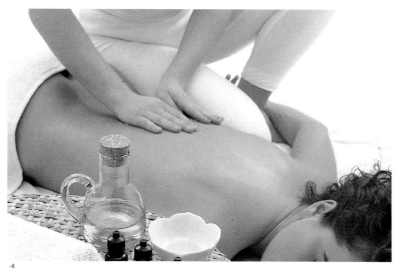

1 Slowly and gently massage in the oil, moving your hands down each side of the spine.

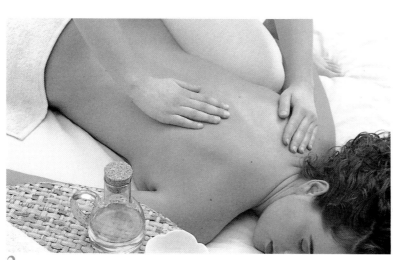

2 For relaxation, use one hand after the other to stroke down the back in a steady rhythm.

If possible, use one of the following blends in a base oil, and get your partner to massage you for the perfect antidote to that overdose of life's stresses.

• For aiding relaxation, 3 drops lavender, 3 drops geranium and 3 drops marjoram.

• For both calming and soothing, as well as giving a gentle uplift, 4 drops rose and 3 drops jasmine.

• For a more definitely uplifting and energizing effect, try 3 drops clary sage and 4 drops bergamot.

Marjoram

Geranium

SENSUAL OILS

Tension, anxiety, worry, depression – all these can affect your sexual energy and performance.
Sometimes this starts a negative spiral of anxiety about sex, leading to less enjoyment and
so on. Take a little time out of your hectic life to be together with your partner and have fun;
add to your sensual pleasure with an intimate massage session, using one of these blends to release
tensions and allow your natural sexual energy to respond.

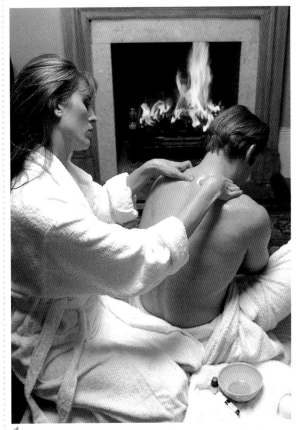

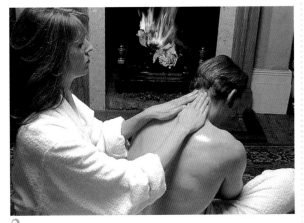

2 Finish the massage with light, caring strokes all
over the body.

Use whichever of these blends – 5 drops rose and
5 drops sandalwood or 4 drops jasmine and 4 drops
ylang ylang – appeals to you both, and include a
massage oil. Use gentle, stroking movements all over
the back, buttocks, legs and front.

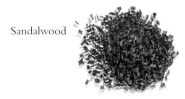

Sandalwood

1 Use firm massage movements to ease out the knots
in the muscles; this will quickly relax your partner.

TRAVEL CALMERS

They say that travel broadens the mind; unfortunately, for some people it contracts the mind into a series of worries – will the car break down? Is this plane safe? Will I be sick? If you are a poor or anxious traveller, try using one of the following essential oils to calm the mind and stomach, letting you enjoy the delights of new horizons without being stressed by how to reach them.

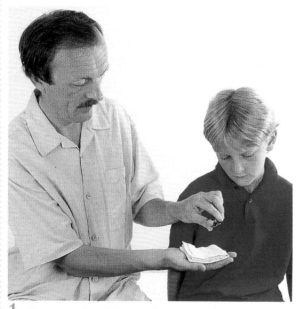

1 Put a couple of drops of essential oil on a tissue.

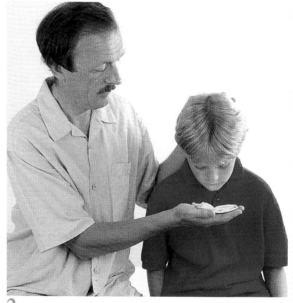

2 Hold the tissue under the nose and lean the head slightly forward. Inhale.

The simplest way to use essential oils when travelling is to put a couple of drops on to a tissue or handkerchief, and smell them frequently. Useful oils are peppermint, mandarin or neroli.

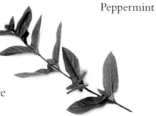

Peppermint

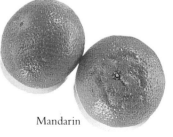

Mandarin

DIGESTIVE SETTLERS

Nervousness often shows itself in an upset stomach, or abdominal spasms. It has been said that our digestive organs also digest stress, and too often they end up storing emotions, causing all manner of discomfort and indigestion. The key is to allow our bodies to let go of such worries and anxieties, and aromatherapy can help a great deal to achieve this. One of the easiest ways to use oils in this context is to make a hot compress and place it over the abdomen, keeping the area warm for up to 10 minutes.

Use a bowl of hot water, with either 2 drops orange and 3 drops peppermint or 3 drops chamomile and 2 drops orange.

Peppermint

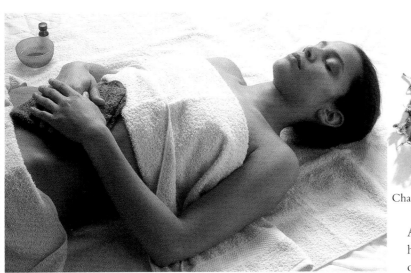

Chamomile

Above: Soak a flannel in a bowl of hot water. Left: Place the compress over the abdomen and relax.

BREATHING ENHANCERS

"Breathe" . . . how often have we said this to ourselves when we are tense and stressed?
Although breathing occurs normally without our conscious control, it can be affected to a
considerable extent as we tense up, tightening the chest muscles and restricting lung expansion.

If you tend to tighten across the chest, try using this aromatic blend as a steam inhalation. To a bowl of steaming water add 3 drops benzoin, 2 drops marjoram and 2 drops eucalyptus.

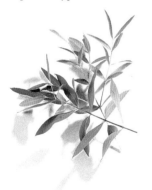

Eucalyptus

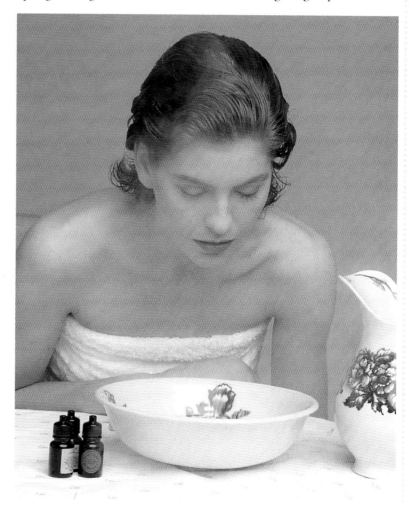

Right: As the oils vaporize, inhale the steam deeply. If you hold a towel over your head this will slow down the evaporation.

CIRCULATION IMPROVERS

A healthy circulatory system is vital to your well-being, both in mind and body. A sluggish circulation will cause a depletion of vital nutrients, leading to exhaustion, ill-health, and even depression. Massage with stimulating essential oils, combined with a healthy diet and exercise, is an excellent way of boosting both blood and lymph circulation in order to promote health and vitality.

For a stimulating massage, create a blend by adding 3 drops black pepper or rosemary to your base oil, plus 2 drops eucalyptus for a detoxifying effect.

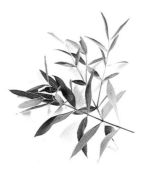

Eucalyptus

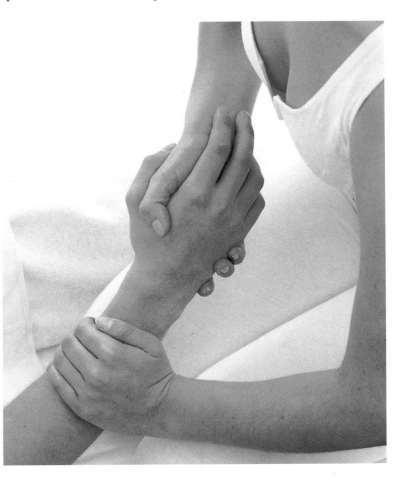

1 The signs of a sluggish circulation include pale, mottled or blue-tinged skin, which is usually cold to the touch. Lift each limb and apply flowing strokes to boost and drain the blood supply on its return to the heart.

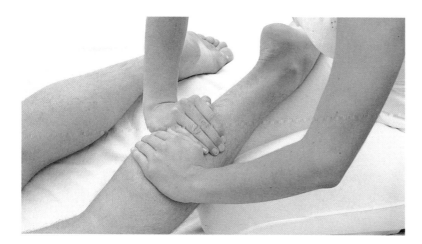

2 Help to increase vitality in the legs and feet by stroking firmly from the ankle to the back of the knee, with the lower leg raised. This position also helps to drain excess water from around puffy ankles.

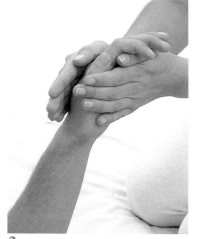

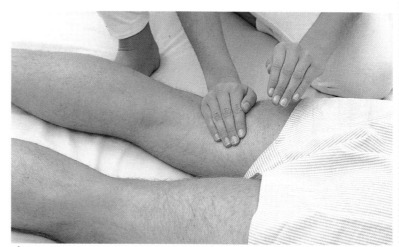

3 Hands and feet that are cold as a result of poor circulation can be warmed up by briskly rubbing them between both hands. The friction produces heat and stimulates the blood supply.

4 Pale, flaccid skin benefits from the stimulating effects of percussion strokes, particularly cupping, which draws the blood up towards the surface of the skin. If the person you are massaging has sensitive skin, a towel can be placed over the legs or buttocks during cupping, this will reduce any stinging sensation but still improve the local blood supply. However, it may be better to carry out lighter cupping movements.

ESSENTIAL OILS FOR COMMON AILMENTS

This chart provides a ready reference to those essential oils that are suitable for use in the home, and some of the more common complaints and disorders they may be used to treat.

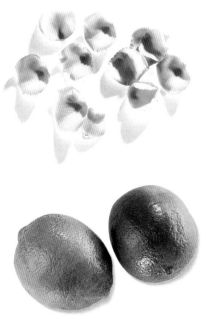

	acne	arthritis	athlete's foot	bad breath	boils, blisters	brittle nails	broken veins	bronchitis, chest infections	bruises	burns	chillblains	cold sores	cystitis, urinary infections	dandruff		
BENZOIN		*						*			*		*			
BERGAMOT	*			*				*				*	*			
BLACK PEPPER		*														
CEDARWOOD	*	*						*					*			
CHAMOMILE	*	*								*	*		*	*		
CLARY SAGE	*				*									*		
CYPRESS								*					*			
EUCALYPTUS		*						*					*			
FENNEL								*	*							
FRANKINCENSE								*					*			
GERANIUM	*								*	*	*		*	*		
GINGER		*						*								
GRAPEFRUIT	*															
JASMINE																
JUNIPER	*	*											*			
LAVENDER									*	*						
LEMON	*	*			*	*		*	*		*	*				
MANDARIN	*															
MARJORAM		*						*	*		*					
NEROLI							*									
NUTMEG		*														
ORANGE																
PALMAROSA	*												*			
PEPPERMINT	*			*												
ROSE							*									
ROSEMARY	*													*		
ROSEWOOD	*															
SANDALWOOD	*												*			
TEA TREE	*		*							*		*	*	*		
YLANG YLANG																

dermatitis	earache	eczema	'flu	heavy periods	hiccups	insect bites	irregular periods	lack of, or late periods	menopause	mouth ulcers, gum infections	neuralgia	nosebleeds	palpitations	period pain	piles (hemorrhoids)	PMS	rashes, allergies	rheumatism	scars	skin ulcers	sore throat, laryngitis	spots	sprains, strains	thrush	warts, verrucas	wounds, cuts, sores
			*							*							*	*					*			*
		*	*			*															*			*	*	*
			*								*							*								
																		*								
	*		*			*			*					*		*	*	*					*	*		
								*						*		*						*				
			*	*					*					*	*			*								
			*			*																				
					*			*	*									*								
			*	*										*				*	*	*	*			*		*
		*					*		*													*	*			*
			*				*											*					*	*		
			*										*													
							*							*				*					*	*		
*		*	*			*								*	*			*								*
	*	*	*			*		*						*				*								*
		*				*					*	*			*		*	*					*	*	*	*
				*																			*			
								*						*	*			*						*		
		*							*	*			*					*								
			*						*																	
*		*											*					*							*	*
*		*											*													
		*					*						*	*						*						
*		*	*	*									*	*				*								
*																								*		*
		*																						*		*
		*				*				*								*					*	*	*	*
													*													

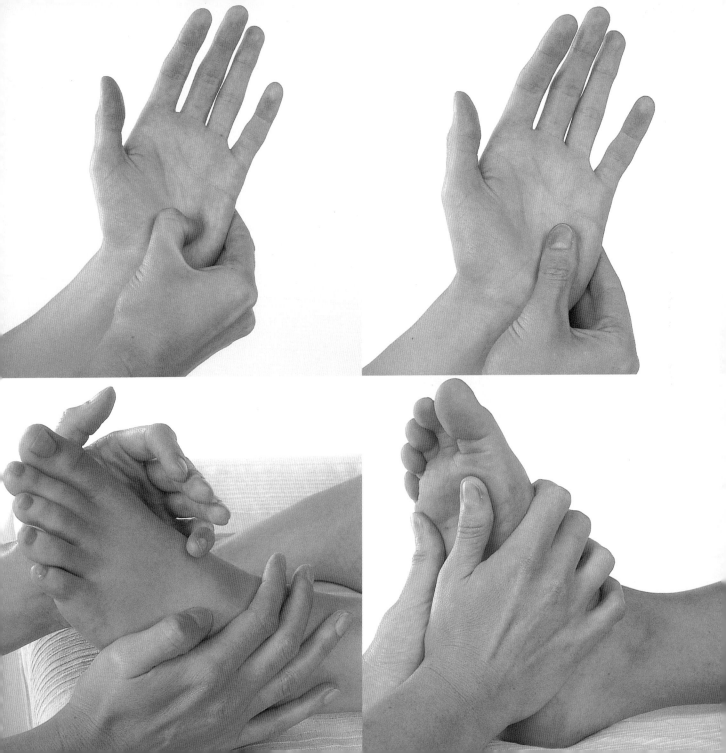

POINTS OF ENERGY: *the Art of Reflexology*

IN PHYSICS – the science of the properties of matter and energy – the behaviour and movement of energy is clearly understood. This applies equally to our bodies, as we are part of the natural world and subject to its laws. In natural medicine the energy within us is known as the life force or vital energy. Reflexology works by using massage to clear away the congestion of toxic deposits that inhibits this flow of energy through our bodies, thus improving our health and vitality.

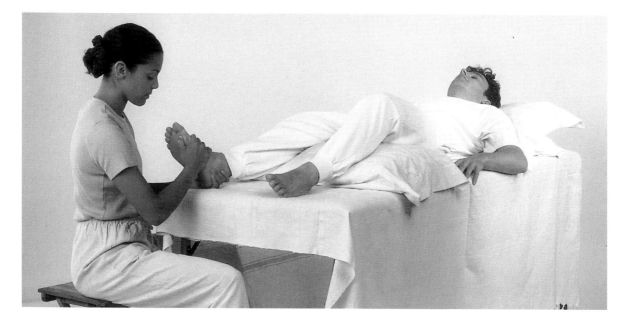

HOW REFLEXOLOGY WORKS

REFLEXOLOGY ACTS ON PARTS OF THE BODY by stimulating the corresponding reflexes with compression techniques applied with the fingers. Where there is inhibited functioning, or disease, we find congestion in the form of deposits that have not been cleared away by the venous circulation and the lymph.

Places on the feet where there are congestion deposits will feel tender, sensitive or positively painful; or they may feel hard, tight or lumpy, or like little grains. If these can be worked with massage and compression techniques so that they begin to disperse, the corresponding body part will be stimulated and enabled to heal itself.

HOW THE BODY FITS ON TO THE FEET

Both feet together hold the reflexes to the whole body. The part that corresponds to the spine therefore runs down the medial line along the instep (the inner edge) of each foot. It will be useful to refer to the charts at the back of the book when reading this section, as they show a picture of the inside body parts in each area of the feet.

Right: Working on the spinal reflex that runs along the instep of each foot.

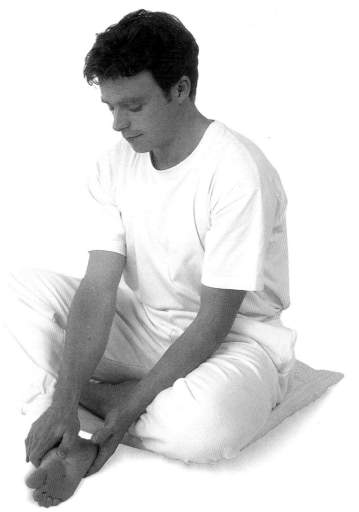

HEAD AND NECK

Your head is represented on the toes; the right side of your head lies on the right big toe and the left side on the left big toe. In addition to the whole head being fully represented on the two big toes, the eight little toes hold the reflexes to specific parts of your head, for fine tuning.

Your neck reflex is found in the "necks" of all the toes: if you find tension in one area of your neck, you will find tension or discomfort, or be able to feel congestion, in the corresponding areas of your toes. The correspondence between the head and toes may be difficult to understand at first because you have only one head and ten toes (or only two sides to your head and five toes on either side).

TORSO AND SPINE

It is much easier to comprehend how the torso fits on to the body of the feet once you have grasped the concept of your two feet together representing your whole body. Remember that the spinal line runs down the insteps of your feet, where they meet if you put them together.

ZONES ON THE FEET

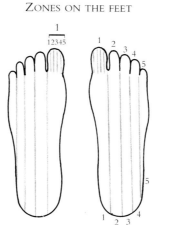

Above: This diagram shows the zones running along the feet. The big toes represent the whole head, as well as lying in Zone 1. The right side of your body lies on your right foot, and the left side of your body on the left foot.

ZONES ON THE BODY

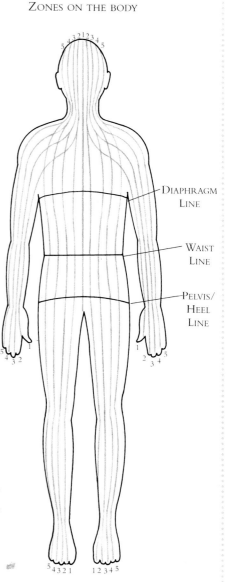

DIAPHRAGM LINE

WAIST LINE

PELVIS/ HEEL LINE

Right: The zones run vertically through the body, from head to feet and hands, five on each side. The diagram also shows the transverse lines marking the areas of the body.

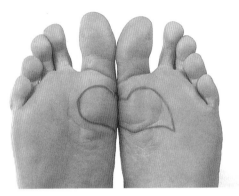

CHEST

The ball of each foot represents one side of your chest. So in the balls of your feet, and on the same area on the top of your feet, lie the reflexes to your lungs, air passages, heart, thymus gland, breast, shoulders and everything contained in your chest. The whole area is bounded by your diaphragm, the important reflex that lies across the base of the ball of each foot.

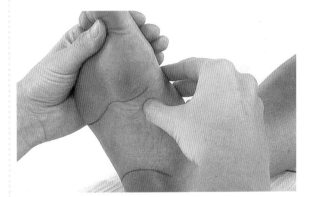

ABDOMEN

In your instep, where your feet are not weight-bearing and so not padded like the ball, are contained all the reflexes to your abdominal organs - those concerned with digestion and the maintenance of life. This area is bounded by the diaphragm line above and by the heel line below.

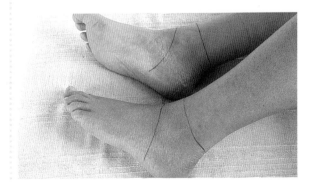

PELVIS

The whole of your heel all around your foot contains the reflexes to your pelvic area: they lie on the sole and the sides of your heel and across the top of your ankle.

LIMBS

The limbs are represented on the outer edge of your foot but also, and most particularly, on the corresponding upper or lower limb. There is no part of the foot that resembles the limbs, whereas you can see fairly easily how the head corresponds to the toes and the torso to the body of the foot. Arms and legs, however, follow the same basic structure and each limb holds the reflexes to the other limb on the same side. These are called cross reflexes.

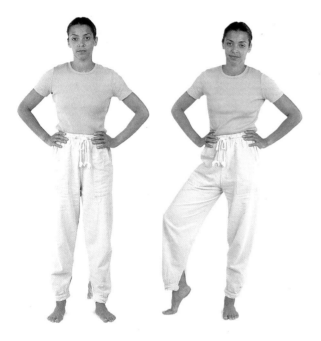

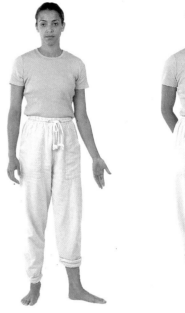

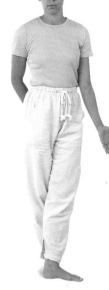

Shoulders reflect hips, and hips reflect shoulders, so you can work your shoulder for hip problems and vice versa.

In the same way, elbows and knees relate to each other.

Work the wrist for ankle problems, and vice versa.

Hand and foot are cross reflexes for each other.

THE BENEFITS AND EFFECTS OF REFLEXOLOGY

Reflexology works to relax muscle tension. During a treatment all parts of the feet are stimulated to relax muscles and increase the circulation to all parts of the body. The immediate effect of this is to achieve a deep state of relaxation.

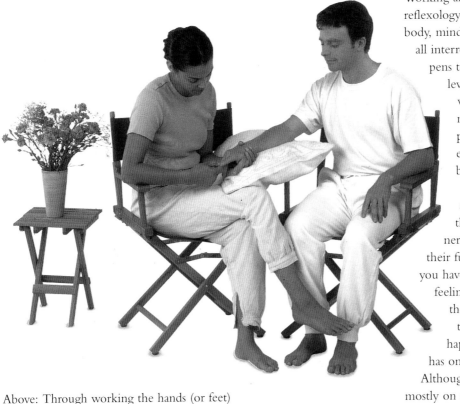

Above: Through working the hands (or feet) you are working the whole body.

Working along holistic principles, reflexology takes into account body, mind and spirit as these are all interrelated. Whatever happens to you will affect all levels of your being, whether you notice or not. If you feel under pressure or stressed, the effect on your body will be detrimental as your muscles remain tense and taut, constricting the circulation and nerves, and compromising their functioning. Similarly, if you have a physical mishap your feelings will be affected by the pain you experience, the way the accident happened, and the effect it has on you afterwards.

Although you are working mostly on the feet in reflexology, you are affecting the whole of the body, both inside and out, through the treatment. This is achieved by working the reflexes to the internal organs and glands as well as to the surface of the body. It appears that you can have a more far-reaching effect by working the reflexes than by working directly on the corresponding body part.

Pain in the back, for instance, may be due to a structural problem in which the bones are actually out of place and should be checked by a cranial osteopath, osteopath or chiropractor. If the pain results from muscular problems, or if manipulation has already been done but muscular strain remains, the next step is to identify the muscles involved and work to relieve the situation with massage and reflexology.

Massage has an immediate and profoundly relieving effect, but the pain and discomfort is likely to recur when the effects of the massage have worn off. Longer term benefits result from working the reflexes to the relevant area of the back than from working directly on those muscles concerned. This is because through the reflexes you are stimulating the body from within, rather than exercising and

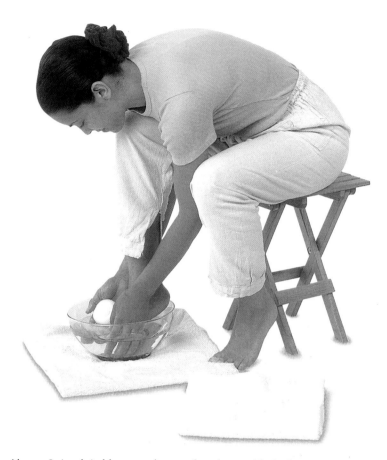

Above: It is advisable to wash your feet thoroughly before any treatment to cleanse and refresh the skin.

soothing the muscles from without. Stimulating the reflex to a troubled area will promote healing. Reflexology uses both massage and specific stimulation of the reflexes to gain lasting relief.

WHAT A TREATMENT INVOLVES
Reflexology is not foot massage, but this is incorporated. Sweeping whole hand movements on the whole foot will relax the entire person and prepare the feet for

reflex work. During the working of the reflexes, massage soothes and relaxes the area where congestion or discomfort is found. It links the treatment together into a continuous whole and relaxes and stimulates the whole body while individual parts are being treated specifically. Equally beneficial is the use of whole hand massage movements to complete a reflexology treatment and to give a feeling of well-being to the entire person before ending the treatment.

A reflexology session can be both relaxing and stimulating for the patient. As muscle tensions are relaxed, and the nerve supply freed from constriction, the body slips into a deep state of relaxation. At the same time, the circulation is being stimulated to bring nutrients to all parts of the body and to remove waste products and toxins that interfere with the healthy functioning of the parts and the whole. Energy is able to flow more freely and fully around the body, the functioning of the various systems is thus optimized and feelings of well-being result.

THE EFFECTS: WHAT YOU MAY FEEL LIKE AFTER REFLEXOLOGY TREATMENT

Some people find that they feel relaxed and sleepy for some time after a reflexology session; they may feel very tired and need to rest for a while. Many others feel deeply relaxed at the end of a session but find that when they leave, or soon afterwards, they feel energized and motivated.

TOXINS AND THE HEALING REACTION

Waste products are formed in the body as a result of muscular activity; others are the result of your intake of processed food, additives, drugs or any other substances that your body recognizes as alien or unwanted. Included in this group of waste products that the body finds toxic are the by-products of stress as well as those of routine muscular processes.

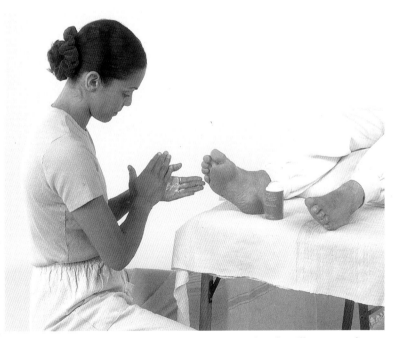

Above: A little powder lightly dusted on to your hands will prevent them from sticking while working on the feet.

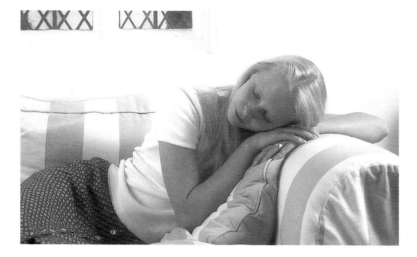

Left: You may feel deeply relaxed after a reflexology treatment.

These healing reactions will pass in hours, or at most in a couple of days, as the body finds a new equilibrium. If, following reflexology, discomfort or illness occurs that does not represent a loosening of the body and evidence of improved functioning, then it is likely to have nothing to do with the treatment and a doctor should be consulted.

Where there are many waste products to be cleared, you may experience a healing reaction (sometimes referred to as a healing crisis) to treatment, which will rid the body or mind of unwanted substances. It may take the form of a runny nose, increased perspiration or urination, or increased bowel movements. You may feel emotional or dream more if the unwanted "substances" are feelings, or even suffer from a headache when feelings can find no other mode of expression. Whatever the reaction, it will be a "throwing off" and will represent a loosening of body tensions and evidence of improved functioning.

CAUTION:

If you choose to use this book to try reflexology yourself, it is imperative that you do so only when the person receiving it is in good health. If you know someone who is ill and who would like to receive reflexology, they should be treated by a recognized and accredited practitioner. A professional reflexologist will never treat someone without first checking on their medical condition and background, and when there is any illness or disorder will advise that the client consult their doctor before proceeding.

If you wish to give reflexology to someone who does not have any medical condition but who does not seem to be well, or who has one of the everyday "first-aid" discomforts described in the sequences in this book, it is again imperative that if they seem at all worryingly unwell they should receive professional help before you do anything at all. If you are subsequently able to give some reflexology you must still proceed with great caution to safeguard both of you from mishap.

PREPARATION

Make sure the room you are going to use is warm and that you may be quiet in there without interruptions from the telephone, people coming in and going out, or restless pets.

Find a comfortable position for the person whose feet you are going to be treating. They may be propped up along a sofa, with cushions to support their back, head and neck in one corner, and their feet at the opposite front edge of the sofa so that you can reach them. If they are sitting in an armchair, find an upright chair or stool of a suitable height to support their legs, with a cushion underneath them. Alternatively, you can position your partner on the floor (see right). Make sure that their back, neck and head are fully supported so as not to place the spine under any strain, and that the knees are bent so that the circulation can flow freely: do not work with the knees straight.

If your partner has sore feet and you are going to work on their hands, it is probably easier to learn the reflexes if you sit side by side rather than opposite each other. In this way the hands will be the same way up as when you are

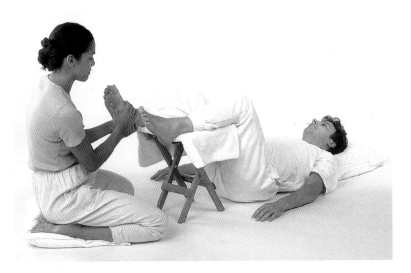

Above: The feet must be where you can comfortably reach them.

Right: Support your arms comfortably while you do reflexology on your hands. Being comfortable will help you to relax.

working on your own hands.

To work on your own feet or hands, find a position that is comfortable for you.

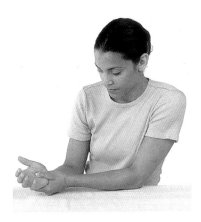

EQUIPMENT

Whichever position you use, you will need to have plenty of pillows to support the back, neck and head. A pillow should be placed under your partner's knees so that they are bent.

Have a blanket or cover ready in case your partner needs extra warmth - their body temperature may drop as they relax.

You will need some towels: one to place under the feet and one or two more for the foot you are not working on to cover it and keep it warm.

Have some powder or arrow-root in case you find that your hands stick to the skin of the feet as you work, if much heat or moisture is released.

Arrange a pile of cushions, a big cushion or a low stool to sit on as you work. You need to be able to reach and see the feet comfortably without bending over from too high above them. It is very important that you are comfortable: becoming strained or tired will not be good for you, and you may not pay attention properly as you work and could risk doing some damage to your partner.

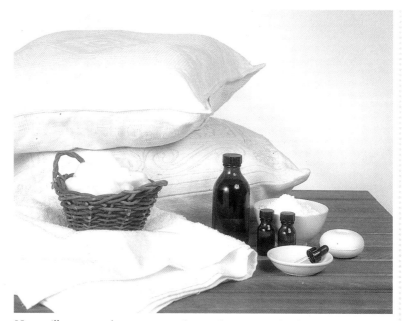

Have pillows, towels, cotton wool, powder, soap and oils handy.

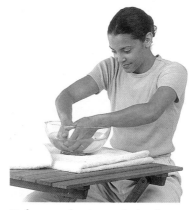

Before you begin, wash the feet or hands in soap and water.

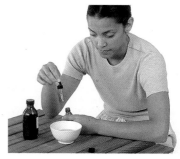

Alternatively, if you have and use essential oils, use a small bowl of water and add a couple of drops of lavender and one of tea tree oil to cleanse them.

WARM-UP FOOT MASSAGE

It is of great benefit to the patient if the feet are massaged at the beginning of a reflexology treatment to introduce your patient to your touch. You should also massage in between specific reflex work, and also to complete the treatment at the end.

TO BEGIN
Massage prepares the feet for reflex work: it warms and relaxes the tissues, accustoms the receiver to your touch and soothes and relaxes the whole body. Massage will loosen tensions in the muscles and stimulate the blood supply to and around the feet so that when the reflex points are worked the tissues will not be strained and they can respond fully.

DURING TREATMENT
Use plenty of massage to link the movement from one reflex area to the next, to soothe and relax the foot in between working the reflex points, which may produce sensations of tenderness, and use it where any tenderness or discomfort is found.

TO COMPLETE
When you have covered all the reflex points, do not just stop, as this could leave your partner feeling fragmented. It is much more pleasant to end with some whole hand massage on both feet to round the treatment off and instil a sense of well-being and relaxation. At this point you may use 2-3 drops of essential oil mixed in almond oil, which will feel flowing and nurturing. Do not use oils in massage until you have completed the reflex work, as your hands will slide around and not be accurate.

THE MASSAGE MOVEMENTS
There is no set sequence for these movements. When you have learnt them, fit them together in a way that feels good to you and adapt them for the individual you are working with as you feel is appropriate. The first few are good as an introduction, and you should always rotate the ankles as this frees up the blood and nerve supply through the ankle to the foot.

EFFLEURAGE OR STROKING

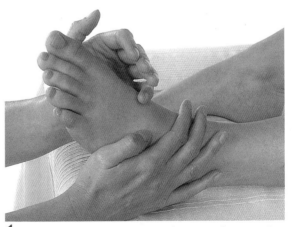

1 These movements are just as they sound - sweeping and soothing - and are good to do all over the foot. Add some effleurage wherever it feels appropriate throughout the treatment.

SPREADING MOVEMENTS

Use these to relax the muscles and stimulate the circulation.

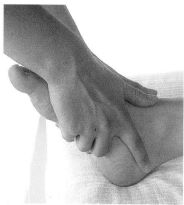

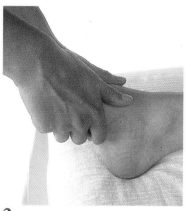

1 For the top of the foot, draw your thumbs off sideways, keeping your fingers still.

2 Repeat the first movement, working your way down the foot with each repetition.

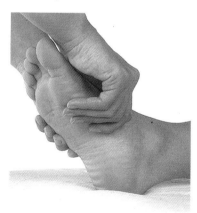

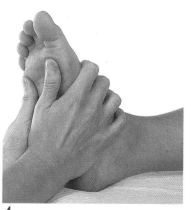

3 To cover the sole of the foot, start in the same position as before, but this time draw your fingers off sideways, keeping your thumbs still.

4 Finally, massage into the ball of the foot with your thumbs.

ANKLE ROTATION

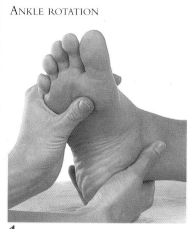

1 Rotate the foot clockwise several times, feeling as you go so that you do not force stiff ankles but you do exercise the joint.

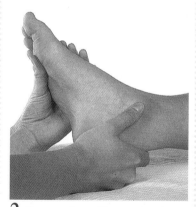

2 Repeat the ankle rotation in an anti-clockwise direction.

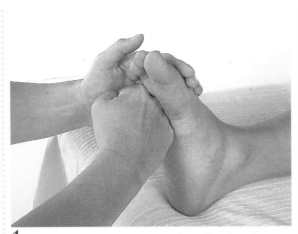

1 Using a similar movement to kneading bread dough, work into the sole of the foot using the lower section of your fingers, not your knuckles. Use your other hand to support the front of the foot, as shown.

VIGOROUS, FAST MOVEMENTS

These are used to stimulate sluggish tissues or help to bring a sleepy person "back to earth" at the end of a treatment. In all these movements your two hands move in opposite directions to one another.

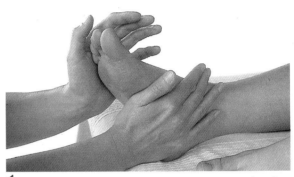

1 Massage the sides of the foot, running your hands up and down the length of the foot.

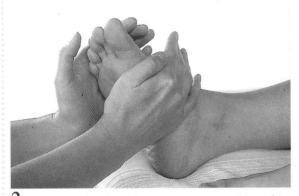

2 With your hands in the same starting position, this time move them alternately up and down from the top to the sole of the foot so that the foot tips from side to side. Take care not to twist the ankle.

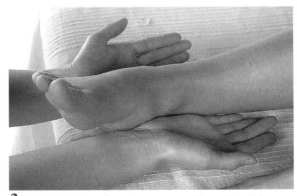

3 With your hands palms up on either side of the foot, move them quickly to and fro, to exercise and loosen the ankle. When this movement is done correctly, the foot will waggle around.

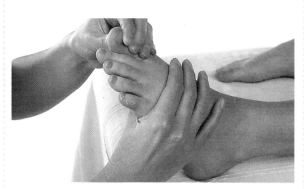

Beginning with the big toe, hold the toe securely (but not too tightly) and gently rotate. Repeat the movement with each toe.

TO RELAX THE DIAPHRAGM

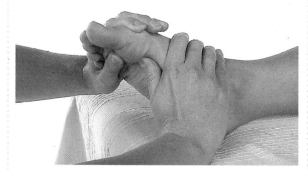

This movement is rather like drawing beer from a traditional hand pump. Hold the foot with your outside hand (the one nearest the little toe), bring the foot down on to the thumb of your other hand and lift it off again. Next, move your thumb one step to the side and repeat the movement. Repeat until you have worked along the boundary line of the ball of the foot where it meets the instep (the diaphragm line).

SPINAL TWIST

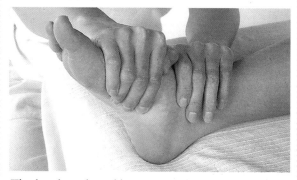

The hand on the ankle remains still while the other, lower hand moves to and fro across the top of the foot, round the instep and back again.

TO ESTABLISH GOOD BREATHING AND RELAX THE SOLAR PLEXUS REFLEX

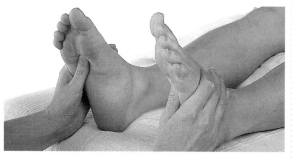

Take both feet together and position your thumbs in the centre of the diaphragm line where there is a natural dent, or place that "gives" when you press gently. Ask your partner to breathe in and then to release the breath. As they breathe in, press gently in with your thumbs and as they breathe out, release your thumbs. Repeat this several times following your partner's lead so that the rhythm is comfortable for them.

REFLEXOLOGY TECHNIQUES

GIVING REFLEXOLOGY

Reflexology works on the whole of the body, stimulating the reflexes to the internal organs, glands and body parts, as well as massaging the outside of the body. Through working on the feet as a whole, healing is stimulated throughout the body rather than just in one part that may well be influenced, or have influence on, other parts or systems. This is what makes the holistic approach of natural medicine so effective.

When you have a problem, natural therapies do not address you as a machine - repairing or replacing the part that does not work, regardless of its purpose in the functioning of the whole - but treat you in your

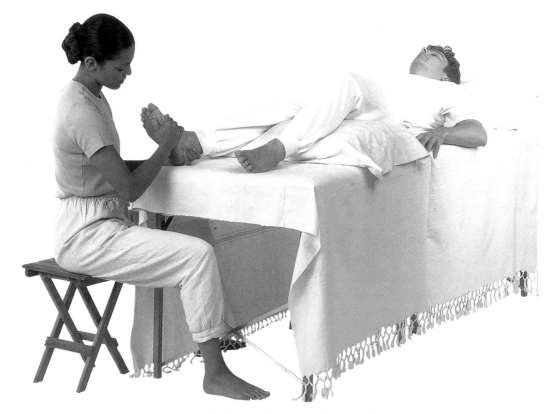

Make sure your partner is comfortable, with pillows under their head, neck and knees acting as support.

entirety to deal with the cause of the problem, rather than merely alleviating the symptoms locally. If you have a raging toothache you may be able to relieve it by taking painkillers, but you will not cause the abscess to go away unless you deal with the poison that gave rise to it in the first place.

If you develop a headache you may or may not know its cause. Where in your body is the trouble seated? Does it come from tension in your neck or lower down your spine, from digestive disturbance, or even from held-in tension in your legs? Many headaches have such roots even though we do not notice the beginning of the trouble until the pounding in our head attracts our attention. Recurrent headaches happen because their causes have not been recognized and dealt with. The headache does not really go away, even if temporarily relieved by taking painkillers.

If you were to gently massage the reflexes to the head you might be able to give temporary relief from the pain, but you will probably not get rid of the headache. Pressing a reflex point for pain relief is helpful, but short-lived. Stimulating a related reflex, usually more than one, which shows congestion or imbalance, on the other hand, is highly effective in the long term. You will only be able to find these if you work the whole of the feet, rather than spot-working for a specific symptom.

In fact, it is quite possible to make a headache worse by stimulating the reflexes to the head, as pressure is already intense there and needs to be relieved lower down, especially on the spinal column, so that it can drain away.

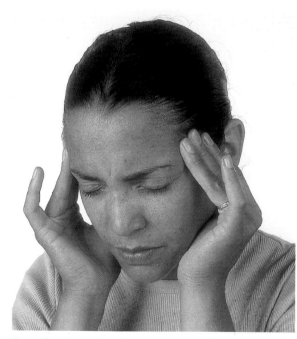

As with a headache, the actual cause of a particular problem may not lie where the pain is located.

CAUTION:

Picking out certain reflexes in isolation is only really effective in the context of working the whole. If you learn and use the routine that follows you will be able to use the sequences in the next section to great effect as part of a reflexology treatment. If you try to bring about a change using only the sequences, you are likely, at best, to be disappointed in the results and, at worst, to aggravate the problem.

FIVE BASIC HAND TECHNIQUES
THUMBWALKING

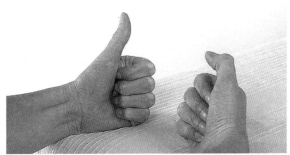

1 Hold your two thumbs straight up in front of you and bend one at a time at the first joint. Thumbwalking is this movement repeatedly performed while the thumb rests on the skin and travels along its surface.

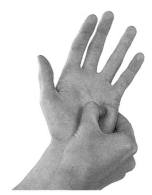

2 The therapeutic movement is on the downward press with your thumb bent. As you press and move forward along the surface, put emphasis on pressing down on the skin. Use one hand only: the other holds and supports the foot or hand you are working on.

ROTATING

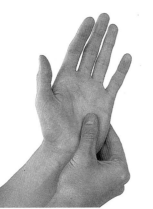

3 Slide or skate forward as you straighten your thumb. You will still put some pressure on the surface and maintain contact but you are primarily involved in moving forward. The thumbwalking technique is sometimes called caterpillar walking.

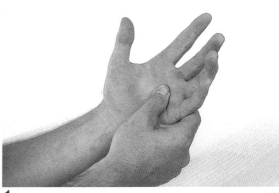

1 Place your thumb (or finger) on a part of your hand or foot and gently rotate it on the spot. Try exerting a little more pressure. Use this technique when you want to work a specific small point.

FINGERWALKING

This technique is the same as thumbwalking, but using one or more fingers.

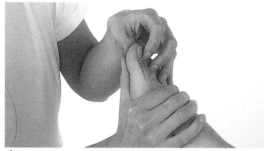

1 Fingerwalking with the index finger.

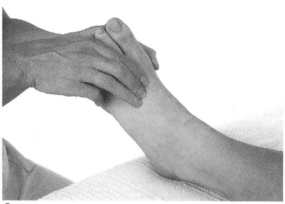

2 Fingerwalking with the three middle fingers together.

PINPOINTING

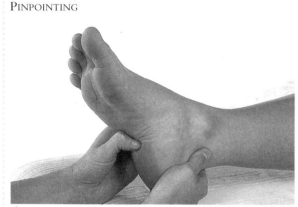

1 Pinpointing is used only for deep or less accessible reflexes that you cannot usually reach by rotating. You use your thumb and fingers in conjunction. With your hand in mid-air, move thumb and fingers together and then apart like a pincer. Now place your hand on the foot or hand and, with the inner corner of your thumb, press deeply down into the tissues. Do this on a well-padded part, or it might hurt the receiver.

HOLDING AND SUPPORT

1 Always use one hand to hold the foot or hand you are working on securely, both to give a feeling of security to your partner and to help yourself to do the techniques properly and sensitively. Position your holding hand near the working hand, not at the other end of the foot, as this can feel insecure.

THE FULL REFLEXOLOGY ROUTINE

The following pages are a step-by-step illustration of the full reflexology routine, which should be performed on your partner before moving to treat specific problem areas. It is good to treat the areas of the body in the same order as outlined here. For easy reference to the areas described, refer to diagram of the routine below. Occasionally, lines have been drawn on the hands and feet in the photographs to highlight key reflex points.

SUGGESTED ORDER FOR REFLEXOLOGY ROUTINE

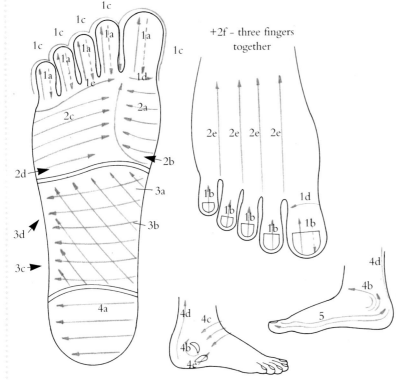

MASSAGE
Remember to begin with some massage and to incorporate massage movements into the whole routine, between every area and when you find a tender place. Give a good thorough massage at the end to complete.

LEFT AND RIGHT
The routine is described for one foot. Begin with the right foot and, when you have completed it, move to the left foot and duplicate what you have done (reversing hands and movements as appropriate to the shape of the left foot). At the end of the routine you will have followed the diagram on both feet. In the diagram (left) each number (ie. area of the body) has subsections marked by letters and the arrows indicate the direction of movement.

This diagram illustrates the order of reflex areas to follow to work the full reflexology routine. Refer to the diagram as often as necessary.

THE SPINE

The spine runs along the instep. Start or finish with this routine.

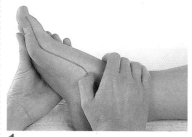

1 Thumbwalk up the spinal line.

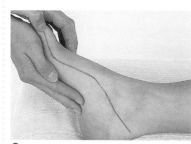

2 Thumbwalk down the spinal line.

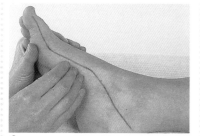

3 Use the three middle fingers to fingerwalk across the spine/instep in stages, from big toe to heel.

THE TOES

The toes refer to the head and neck.

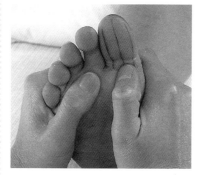

1 Work up the back of the big toe, thumbwalking it in three lines, to cover the whole area.

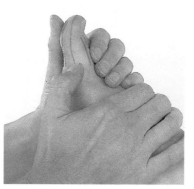

3 Next, work up the side of the big toe with your thumb.

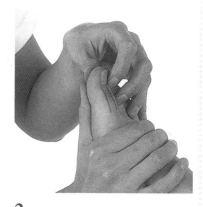

2 Using your index finger, fingerwalk down the front of the big toe, again in three lines.

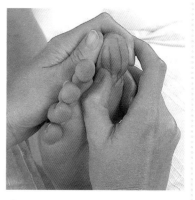

4 For the other side of the toe, approach it from the back and tuck your thumb in between this toe and the second one before you start to thumbwalk the line up the side of the neck. ▶

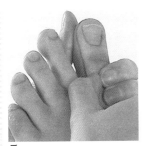

5 Change hands and, using your other thumb, approach from the front and tuck it in between the big toe and second toe again. Work up this side to the top.

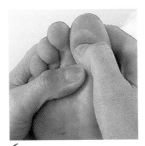

6 Find the centre of the whorls of the big toe print and position your hand for pinpointing the pituitary reflex here. Press gently at first, as it can be tender. If you get no response, check that you are in the centre of the toe print and then press harder, then release.

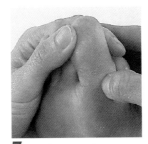

7 Work around the neck of the big toe in two semi-circles: thumb-walk the back first.

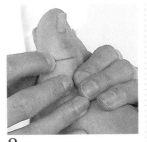

8 Fingerwalk around the front of the big toe, using your index finger.

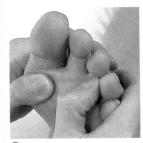

9 For the smaller toes, follow the same routine as for the big toe. These toes can be covered in one line to each surface. Thumbwalk up the back.

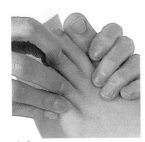

10 Fingerwalk down the front of each toe to its base.

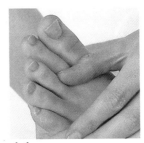

11 Thumbwalk up one side of the toe. Always approach the side from the front. Change hands and work up the other side of the same toe.

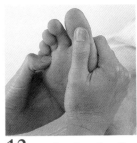

12 Finally, thumbwalk the ridge under the little toes.

THE CHEST

The chest area is contained on the ball of the foot and on the top of the foot.

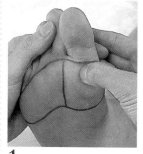
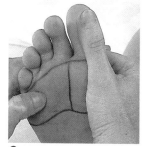
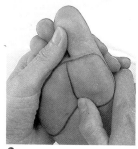
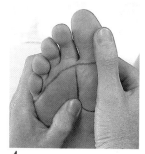

1 Thumbwalk horizontally in from the instep under the big toe in zone 1 (for the five zones, see the illustrations on the head, neck and torso zones in the How Reflexology Works section), starting just next to the neck. Repeat just below the first line, bordering on it. Continue thumbwalking lines like this until you have covered the ball under the big toe down to the diaphragm line.

2 Thumbwalk horizontally in from the outside of the foot under the little toes, starting just below the ridge. Cover the whole of this area in the same way as described in step 1.

3 Next work along the diaphragm line under the big toe and follow the natural line up between the big and second toes to the base of the toes.

4 Work along the diaphragm line from the outside, and when you meet the line between the big and second toes continue up this line to the base of the toes.

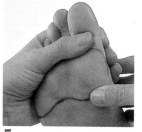
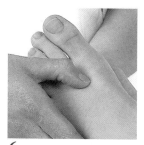
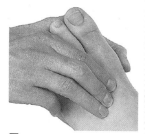

5 Starting from just under the big toe, thumbwalk the whole diaphragm line.

6 On the top of the foot, fingerwalk each channel between the bones leading to the toes.

7 Use the three middle fingers together to fingerwalk the whole of the top of the foot, working from the base of the toes up the foot.

THE ABDOMEN

This area lies in the instep, starting under the diaphragm line and going down to the heel line.

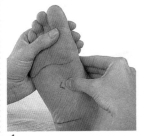

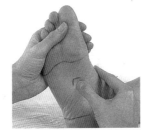

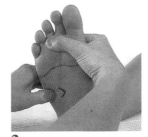

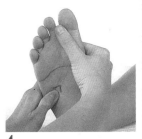

1 Thumbwalk from the medial edge, under the big toe, out to the outer edge in horizontal lines as you did for the chest, each line bordering the previous one.

2 Next thumbwalk diagonal lines covering the same area, as described in step 1.

3 Now change hands and thumbwalk horizontal lines from the outside of the foot to the inner (medial) edge, as before.

4 Finally, with the same thumb, thumbwalk diagonal lines from the outside to the inner edge covering the whole area, as before.

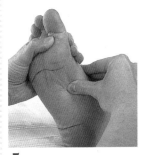

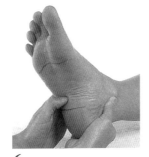

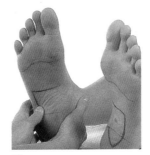

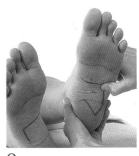

5 Referring to the foot chart at the back of the book, gently rotate the reflex to the adrenal glands, pushing in under the tendon running down from the big toe.

6 Work the ileo-caecal valve reflex, using the inner corner of your thumb to pinpoint it.

7 Thumbwalk the path of the colon, starting on the right foot at the bottom of the colon line.

8 Continue on to the left foot, following the line as outlined on the foot chart at the back of the book. Change from left hand to right hand at the point above.

THE PELVIS

The pelvic area lies all around the heel: on the sole, the sides of the heel and on top of the ankle.

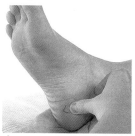

1 Thumbwalk the heel across the sole in horizontal, overlapping lines. (This is hard work.)

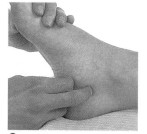

2 Find the little hollow halfway along a diagonal line between the centre of the ankle bone and the right angle of the heel on the inside of the foot, and rotate this point with your middle fingertip. Do not apply too much pressure.

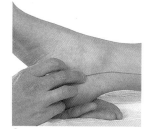

3 From this point, fingerwalk with the same finger up the line running behind the ankle up the leg.

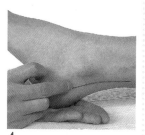

4 Now find the point described in step 2, but on the outside of the foot. Rotate it with the middle finger of your other hand and then fingerwalk up the outside of the ankle and leg, just as you did on the inside.

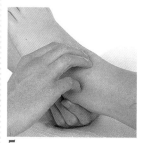

5 Using the three middle fingers, fingerwalk across the top of the ankle.

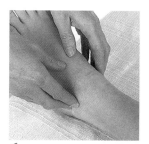

6 Continue round the ankle bone with the same fingertips.

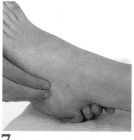

7 Refer to the foot charts to find the hip/knee reflex, and work it by fingerwalking two fingers together.

THE LIMBS

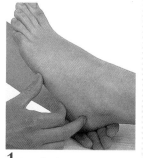

1 Work the outside of the foot, then massage the relevant cross reflex.

THE SEQUENCES

When you have learnt, and feel comfortable with, the whole routine for giving reflexology you may begin to pay special attention to certain reflexes for specific reasons, as you work. Always work the reflex on both feet unless the right or left foot is specified.

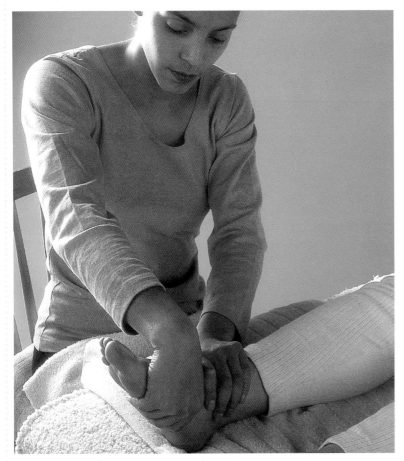

When giving reflexology you must always be sensitive to the response, particularly to painful or congested areas.

HOW TO USE THE SEQUENCES WITHIN THE WHOLE ROUTINE

If you are giving reflexology at the end of the day, for instance, to relax someone and promote a good night's sleep, when you get to the reflex for the diaphragm you will be aware that it is particularly beneficial to work that part in order to assist relaxation and rest, and so you will work with special awareness and sensitivity there.

In giving special attention to certain reflexes you may feel drawn to do more massage in that place, or you may find the reflex is tender and you need to work more gently and perhaps for a little longer to release some of the tension felt there. Or you may stop to rotate on the reflex gently where you would otherwise simply have covered the area by thumbwalking.

Your way of working must be dictated by the response of your partner, taking into account how they feel, how they are experiencing the massage and what they and you can feel on their feet.

WHAT TO DO IF YOUR PARTNER FEELS IT IS PAINFUL

Finding congestion or tenderness on the reflexes is never a reason for enthusiastic working at a specific reflex for an extended period, and you must never ever work if you are causing pain. In this situation massage gently, instead of thumbwalking, and then, if you are able to continue on the tender spot without causing discomfort, do so by working more gently to ensure that you do no harm. The golden rule is that you always take your lead from the person you are working with: follow what they are telling you about where they hurt and where they can take more or less of your touch.

Do not go to the other extreme and miss out parts that hurt, however, as they are just the places that need anything which will assist or stimulate them to heal themselves. Your job is to work out how best you may assist this process and if this means that all you can do without causing pain and discomfort is to hold the

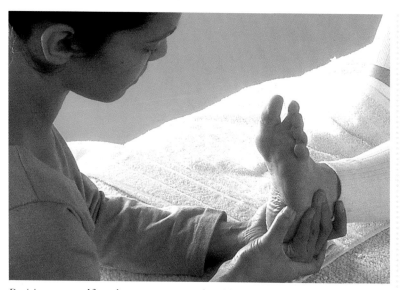

Position yourself so that you are comfortable and have a good view of the soles of the feet.

troubled part gently, or just stroke it with a fingertip, do so.

As long as you listen to your partner, to what they say and to their body language, and take your approach from what they and their feet are telling you, you will be doing well.

If you have not yet read the introduction to this section please read it now before going any further, to make sure that you do no harm. Your treatment of the feet will stimulate and balance all the body systems and you are now

ready to incorporate the sequences that follow, if you wish to highlight specific areas.

CAUTION:
Working any of the following sequences in isolation, without working the whole foot routine, will not be effective and may cause damage. These sequences are for you to add to the basic routine as you work through it.

RELAXATION SEQUENCES
AIDING RESTFUL SLEEP

You will benefit more from a night's sleep if your body is relaxed and tense muscles loosened before you go to bed. Otherwise you may wake stiff, in pain, with a headache or unrefreshed; or you may wake during the night and be unable to get back to sleep.

Through massage and stimulating the reflexes you will improve the circulation and this, in turn, will accelerate the body's removal of waste. In this way you are doing what you can to enhance the systems of the body and to enable it to make the most of the healing properties of sleep.

It is important to use plenty of massage on your partner's feet during the routine. Always include ankle rotation, as this loosens tension there. All the blood supply and nerves to the feet pass through the ankles, and so it is very important that these flow freely, unrestricted by excessive tension.

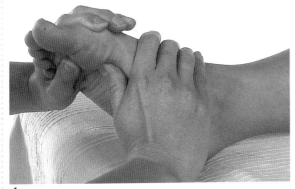

1 To relax the diaphragm, hold the foot with your outside hand, bring it down on to the thumb of your other hand and lift it off again. Move your thumb one step to the side and repeat the movement, until you have worked your thumb across the foot to the outer side, following the boundary line of the ball of the foot where it meets the instep (the diaphragm line).

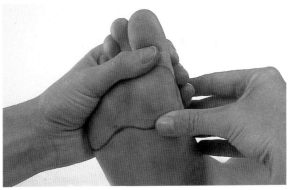

2 Thumbwalk along the whole of the diaphragm line. Relaxing the diaphragm is especially important, as it helps to relax the whole body and to steady breathing.

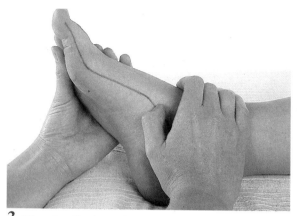

3 Thumbwalk along the spinal reflex from the heel to the big toe. Always remember to support the foot. In this instance, support the outside of the foot with your other hand.

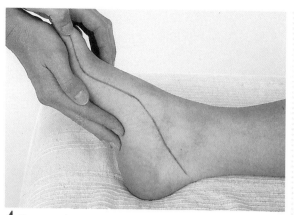

4 Repeat the movement, going down the spinal reflex. Repeat up and down several times. Slow down to feel for any tight or sensitive parts and rotate gently around those spots.

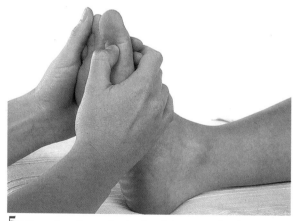

5 Thumbwalk up the back of the toes: do this with care as there is likely to be a lot of tenderness there.

SELF-HELP:

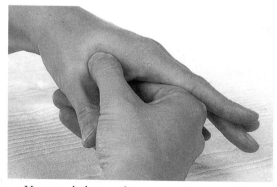

You can help to relax tension in yourself by massaging the web between your thumb and index finger on both hands.

NECK AND SHOULDER RELAXERS

We collect much tension in our necks. If you are not aware of neck tension put your hands on either side of your neck and massage gently. If it feels tight or uncomfortable you may benefit from this sequence as your partner works your feet.

When neck muscles are tense and tight they constrict the nerves, which may in turn lead to pain, noises in the ears, or tired eyes. If you suffer from aching shoulders you will find that relaxing the tense shoulder muscles will not only relieve the aching but will improve your breathing as well. Tight shoulder muscles will pull your chest tight and consequently restrict your breathing.

Within the framework of the whole routine you may pay special attention to the following areas.

NECK TENSION

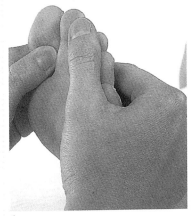

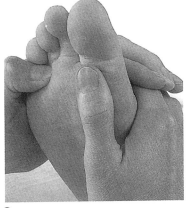

SELF-HELP:

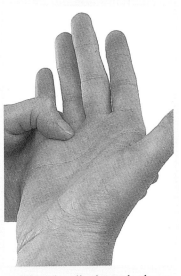

1 Thumbwalk up the side of the neck on the big toe, where a lot of tension collects. Repeat this up the neck of all the toes and thumbwalk around the neck of the big toe, starting from the back.

2 Thumbwalk along the ridge immediately under the toes. Make sure you are right on top of this ridge, as it is easy to move below it, which will not have the same effect.

Thumbwalk along the base of your fingers.

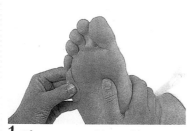

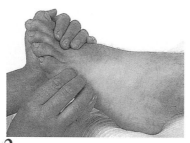

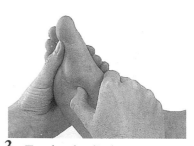

1 If you are working with someone who has shoulder tension, thumbwalk along the line of the shoulders in horizontal, overlapping lines.

2 Fingerwalk across the same area on the top of the foot with three fingers. Then fingerwalk around the mid-back with three fingers, working in rows from the lower joint of the little toe down to the waistline (halfway down the foot).

3 To relax the diaphragm, position your thumb on the diaphragm line underneath the big toe. Hold the foot with your outside hand, bring it down on to the thumb of your other hand and lift it off again. Move your thumb one step to the outer side of the foot and repeat the movement, until you have worked your thumb across the foot to the outer side, following the boundary line of the ball of the foot where it meets the instep (the diaphragm line).

SELF-HELP:
Thumbwalk and massage around the shoulder line on your hands (refer to the hand chart at the back of the book).

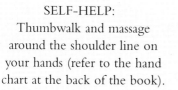

WHIPLASH INJURIES

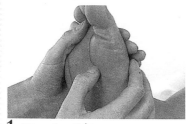

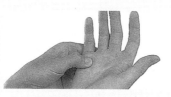

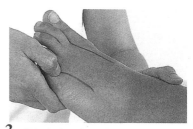

1 Thumbwalk the first channel, between the big and second toes.

2 Work the same area on the top of the feet with your thumb.

3 Work the shoulder reflex on the top and the bottom of the feet.

BACKACHE RELIEVERS

Backache is draining, both from the constant aching and because it saps your strength as it constricts your central nervous system (in the spinal cord). More working days are lost through backache than from any other cause. Release tension and relax the supporting muscles in the following areas.

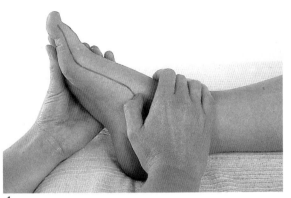

1 Thumbwalk up and down the spine, supporting the outer edge of the foot as you work.

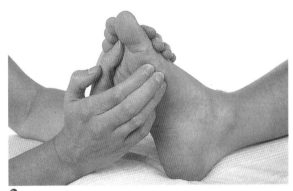

2 Fingerwalk across the spinal reflex with three fingers together, right down the instep in stripes.

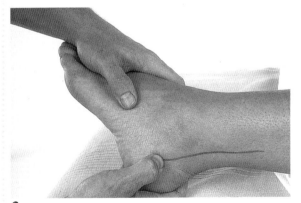

3 Thumbwalk up the helper reflexes for the lower back, behind the ankle bones on either side.

SELF-HELP:

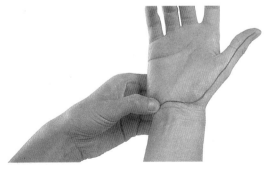

Work the spinal reflex on your hands.

RELIEVING REPETITIVE STRAIN

If you work at a computer for long periods you may suffer from eye strain, or your wrists may ache and hurt from using the keyboard. Any desk job may give you stiff shoulders and a stiff neck. If you are on your feet all day you may well end the day with tired and swollen legs and ankles, and sore feet. The best way to relieve all this strain is to work the whole feet so that the various systems will be stimulated to function more efficiently. In addition you can choose whichever of the following are appropriate.

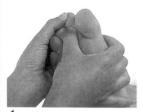

1 Thumbwalk up the back and sides of the second and third toes for the eye reflex. This will also relieve neck tension.

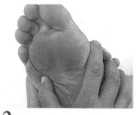

2 Work the shoulder reflexes thoroughly by using the thumbwalking technique.

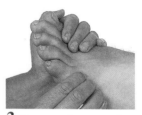

3 Fingerwalk across the same area on the top of the foot, with the three middle fingers together.

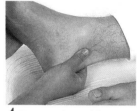

4 Rotate the ankles to ease aching wrists and stimulate healing within the joints.

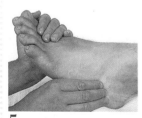

5 Work across and down the outer foot on both feet to relax shoulders, arms, legs and knees.

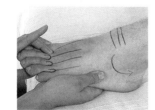

6 Work the lymph system on both feet. Fingerwalk down the lines from the toes towards the ankle. Then work around the ankle.

SELF-HELP:
Use the hand chart at the back of the book to find the relevant reflex on your hands to give temporary, quick relief for your particular problem. The point to remember when dealing with repetitive strain is that there is no one sequence of movements to help. It is up to you to work out which part of your body is suffering from the strain and locate the relevant reflex from the hand and foot charts that are located at the back of the book.

INVIGORATING MUSCLES

Rather than going from one extreme to another and trying to compensate for a sedentary job by doing vigorous exercise with a sluggish body, get someone to give you a foot treatment stimulating the circulation and all the bodily systems. You may then really feel like doing something energetic the next day, because you will feel so much better. You will also benefit more from exercise if your body is not being forced. If you are doing this for someone else, concentrate on the following areas in your full treatment.

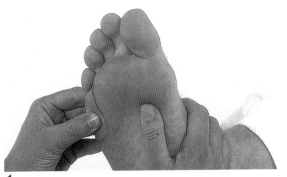

1 Thumbwalk along the line of the shoulders.

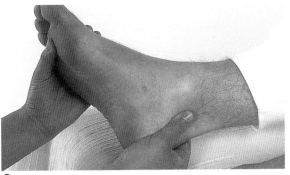

2 Rotate the ankles to loosen tension and increase the circulation and to ease pressure on the nerve supply.

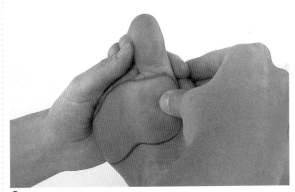

3 Work the whole of the chest and lung area.

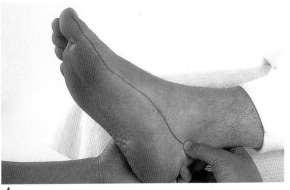

4 Thumbwalk up and down the spine.

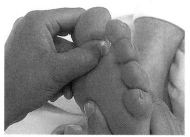

5 Starting with the big toe, work the neck on all the toes.

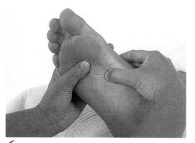

6 Rotate the adrenal reflex gently. This will stimulate it to respond as your body's natural sense directs: to relax and aid recovery from overwork or to stimulate in readiness for activity.

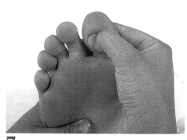

7 Rotate or massage gently on all the reflexes to other important endocrine glands, which regulate the chemicals in your body and therefore your bodily activity.

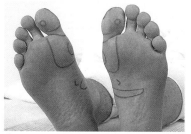

8 Pinpoint the pituitary reflex in the big toe. Thumbwalk the thyroid helper on the ball of the foot. Rotate the adrenals and work the pancreas on the instep.

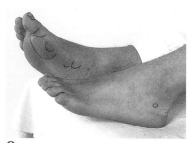

9 Rotate on the ovaries/testes reflex at the side of the heel.

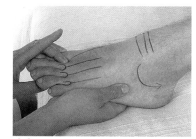

10 Thumbwalk or rotate (as appropriate) the reflexes of the lymph system.

STRESS RELIEVERS

Excessive stress lies somewhere behind most troubles and illness. If your adrenalin runs at a high level for long periods, with little chance of appropriate action, your adrenal glands will become depleted. Your breathing will either become too rapid or will be restricted and shallow. Your digestion will be upset or strained in some way. If you feel nervous or queasy the first thing to do is to breathe more deeply and slowly. This will calm you down, settle your nerves and increase the supply of oxygen to your body. It is not possible to panic while you are breathing well. Help the calming process by working on your hands, massaging with your thumb the solar plexus reflex in your palms. Do this on both hands. If you are giving a reflexology treatment pay special attention to the following areas.

RELIEVING GENERAL STRESS

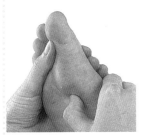 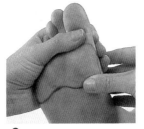 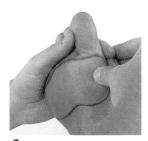 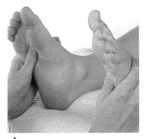

1 Relax the diaphragm: hold the foot with your outside hand, bring it down on to the thumb of your other hand and lift it off again. Move your thumb one step to the outer side and repeat the movement, until you have worked your thumb across the foot, following the boundary line of the ball of the foot.

2 Thumbwalk along the diaphragm line. Tension collects in the diaphragm, causing pain and tightness. When the diaphragm is contracting and relaxing freely the abdominal organs are stimulated also.

3 Work the lung reflexes on the chest area so that once the diaphragm is relaxed, breathing can be increased. This will help you to relax, get the oxygen you need and promote well-being.

4 Do the solar plexus breathing exercise: take both feet together and position your thumbs in the centre of the diaphragm line. As your partner breathes in, press in with your thumbs, and release as they breathe out. Repeat several times following your partner's lead so that it is a comfortable rhythm for them.

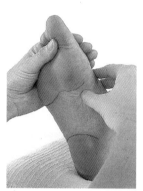 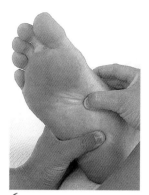 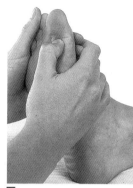 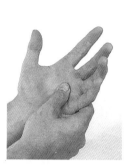

5 Thumbwalk the stomach area and the whole of the instep, which is the abdominal area. This will help digestion and elimination, which are both affected by stress.

6 Rotate gently on the adrenal reflex.

7 Work the neck reflex on the neck of the toes where stress and tension collect.

Massage the centre of your palms, including the solar plexus reflex.

NERVOUS STOMACH OR "BUTTERFLIES"
Work the self-help areas illustrated above right, or steps 4 and 5 for someone to whom you are giving a full treatment.

STRESS FROM ANGER

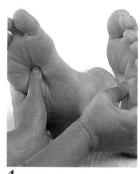 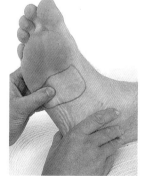

1 Work the solar plexus reflexes on both feet.

2 Work the liver area.

SELF-HELP:
Referring to the hand charts at the back of the book, work the solar plexus reflexes and the liver area on your hands for self-help.

Enhancing Sequences

If you have not yet read the introduction to the sequences please read it now, before you begin, to make sure that you do no harm. Within a treatment covering the whole of the feet, and so stimulating all the bodily systems, you may choose to pay special attention to the following specific areas.

Starting the Day: Stimulating the Systems and the Senses

To make the most of your potential, your bodily systems need to be functioning well as you start the day and to continue to do so throughout the day.

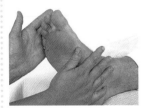 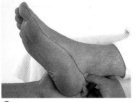 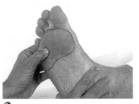 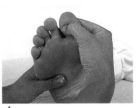

1 Give some good vigorous massage to the whole feet to get the circulation going. Massage the chest area especially to help establish good breathing. Massage the instep using effleurage to stimulate the nervous system in the spinal cord and "wake up" the spine and its supporting muscles.

2 Thumbwalk the spine. Rotate the ankles and the toes to stimulate the circulation to the feet and loosen the neck and pelvis, thus freeing the nerves to the head and lower body.

3 Work the diaphragm, and then work across the chest. This will help to establish deep and regular, steady breathing to strengthen your body.

4 Work the pituitary reflex on the big toe in the centre of the toe-print: this is the master gland and its functioning controls the other endocrine glands and your bodily systems in many ways.

SELF-HELP:

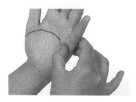

1 To get yourself going at the beginning of the day, work the diaphragm on your hands.

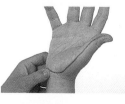

2 Work the spine. Finally, work the pituitary reflex, which is located in the centre of your thumb-print.

IMPROVING DECISIVENESS

When your body is tired and functioning below par, getting through normal daily tasks and making decisions will often seem more difficult. The liver and gall bladder work together so that the body may be strong and planning and decision-making happen naturally. By working the diaphragm, solar plexus and liver you are enhancing good breathing and strengthening the body.

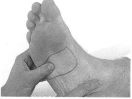

1 Work the liver.

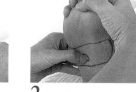

2 Work the gall bladder.

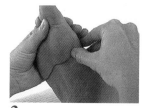

3 Work the diaphragm.

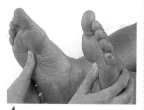

4 Work the solar plexus.

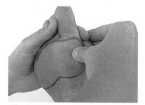

5 Work the lungs.

SELF-HELP:
Locate the gall bladder reflex on your right hand and rotate on it to aid decisiveness.

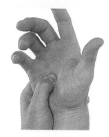

ENERGY LEVEL ENHANCERS

If energy is flowing freely around your body you will feel well and find it easier to feel positive. In turn, if you think positively your body will respond and its actions will be enhanced. The power of thought influences your physical well-being and, conversely, your moods are much affected by your hormonal balance and the general well-being of your body.

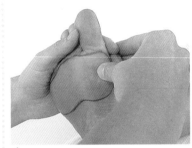

1 Work the lungs to improve your breathing.

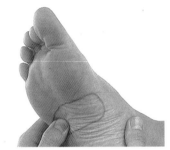

2 Work the liver, the many functions of which are crucial to your general health.

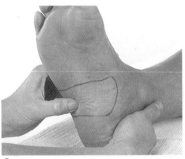

3 Work the small intestines to aid the uptake of nutrients.

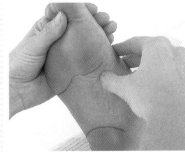

4 Work the whole digestive area. What you eat is turned into your energy during digestion.

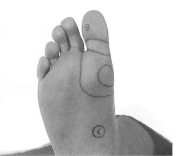

5 Work the glands. Find the pituitary gland on the big toe. Work the thyroid on the neck of the big toe and the ball under it. Rotate the adrenals.

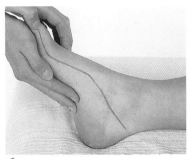

6 Work up and down the spine, which is your central column of energy flow.

SELF–HELP:

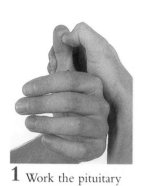 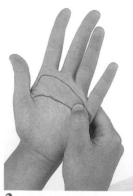 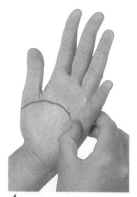

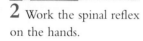

1 Work the pituitary reflex in the centre of the thumb-print.

2 Work the spinal reflex on the hands.

3 Work the lungs to enhance breathing.

4 Work the diaphragm on the hands.

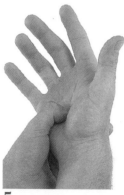 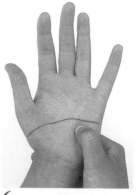 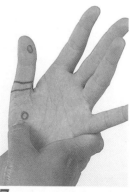

5 Work the liver reflex on your right hand.

6 Work the small intestines.

7 Work the main glands to balance the hormonal system.

IMPROVING SKIN, HAIR AND NAIL CONDITION

To keep your skin, hair and nails in good condition you need hormone balance, good nutrition and effective removal of toxins through the excretory system. Stimulation of the circulation through giving a whole reflexology treatment will aid the removal of toxins from the body and the supply of nutrients through the bloodstream; but remember that the supply of nutrients to your body will only be as good as those you put in through the food you eat. Good health is only possible if you eat a well-balanced mixture of good, "live" food. Poor health will result from processed food which is precooked and then reheated as it has little quality in it.

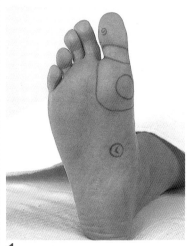

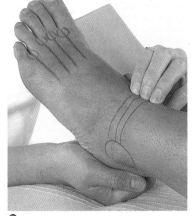

SELF-HELP:

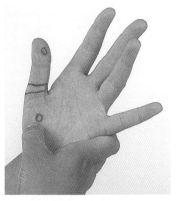

1 Work all the glands on both feet. Your skin, hair and nails are kept in good health by chemicals in your hormones, which are controlled by your glands.

2 In addition, make sure that you give attention to the lymph system on both feet to help remove toxins from the body.

Work all the glands on your hands by referring to the hand chart at the back of the book.

STRENGTHENING THE IMMUNE SYSTEM

Where the immune system is strong, the body will deal naturally with threatening infections so that they cannot become established. Within the context of a full reflexology routine, pay particular attention to the following areas.

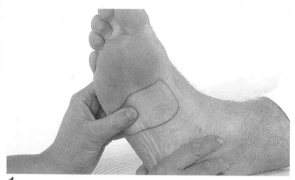

1 Work the liver to strengthen the whole body.

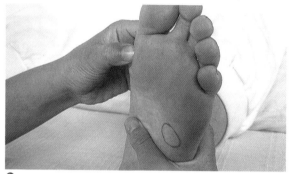

2 Work the spleen (marked on the left foot) and rotate the thymus gland (on both feet) where the thumb is positioned in the above photograph.

SELF-HELP:

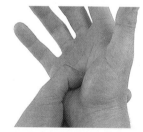

Work the liver and spleen to strengthen your body, and the thymus and lymph to fight off imminent infection. See the hand chart at the back of the book.

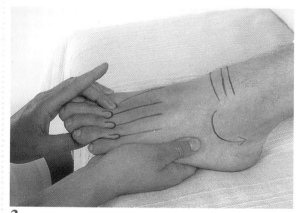

3 Work the upper and lower lymph systems on both feet to aid the removal of toxins.

Relieving Sequences

If you have not yet read the introduction to the sequences please read it now, before you go any further, to make sure that you do no harm. Within a treatment covering the whole of the feet, and so stimulating all the bodily systems, you may choose to pay special attention to the following areas.

Pain Relievers

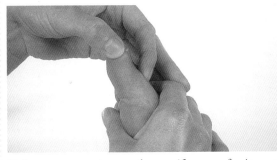

Before concentrating on the specific area of pain, work the hypothalamus reflex: the hypothalamus controls the release of endorphins for the relief of pain.

PAINFUL MUSCLES OR JOINTS

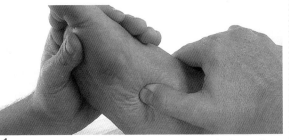

1 Work the adrenal gland reflexes on both feet. These glands deal with inflammation and aid good muscle tone when working effectively.

BACK PAIN

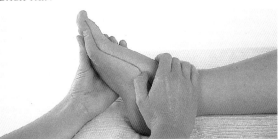

1 Work along the spine and find the tender parts. Work these to try to disperse some of the congestion.

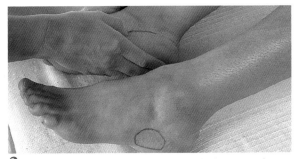

2 For lower back trouble, work the helper area for this by rotating with your thumb.

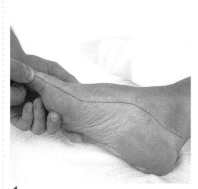

1 Thumbwalk along the spine for the central nervous system in the spinal cord.

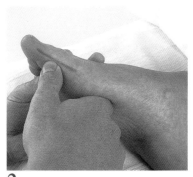

2 Find the local area: for example, for the neck, work the cervical vertebrae and find the part of the neck of the toes that is tender.

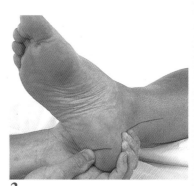

3 For sciatic pain, work the sciatic reflex as shown in the foot chart at the back of the book.

CRAMP

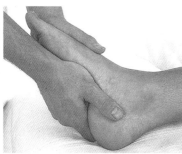

1 Hold the area and massage the appropriate cross reflex. For example, for cramp in the calf, massage the cross reflex on the lower arm.

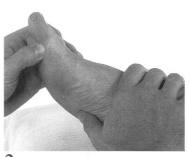

2 Work the parathyroid reflexes round the neck of the big toe.

TOOTHACHE

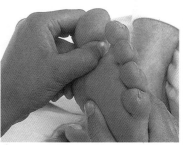

1 Find the toe or finger that has much tenderness and work that area carefully but thoroughly.

SLEEP ENHANCERS

There are many different reasons for insomnia and different manifestations of it. Do you have difficulty in getting to sleep or do you wake during the night and find you cannot get back to sleep? Do you feel the trouble is digestive or are you a worrier? (These two problems may be linked.)
You can help to promote a good night's sleep with this sequence.

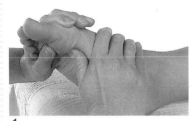

1 To relax the diaphragm hold the foot with your outside hand, bring it down on to the thumb of your other hand and lift it off again. Move your thumb one step to the side and repeat the movement, until you have worked your thumb all the way across the foot to the outer side, following the diaphragm line.

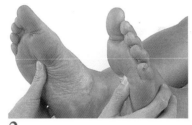

2 Do the solar plexus breathing exercise: take both feet together and position your thumbs in the centre of the diaphragm line. As your partner breathes in, press gently in with your thumbs, and, as they breathe out, release. Repeat this several times following your partner's lead so that it is a comfortable rhythm for them.

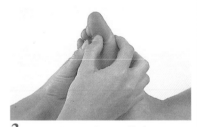

3 Work the neck on all the toes to remove any tension that has built up in the neck muscles.

SELF-HELP:

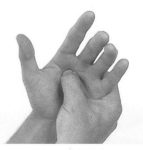

For self-help gently massage the solar plexus reflex in the palms of your hands.

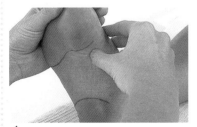

4 Work the abdominal reflexes to relieve tension there.

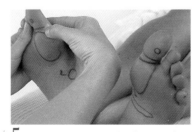

5 Work all the glands, for good hormonal balance.

BREATHING RELIEVERS

Respiratory problems may include hayfever and other allergic reactions. Poor diet, pollution, excessive toxins in the body and excessive stress all undermine the body's strength and may cause a problem in the respiratory system.

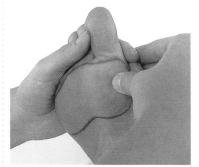

1 Work the whole chest area on bottom of the feet to relieve the chest and lungs.

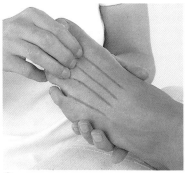

2 Fingerwalk the same area on the top of the feet to stimulate the chest lymph.

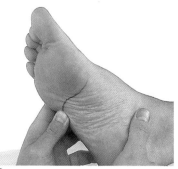

3 Work the diaphragm to promote good breathing.

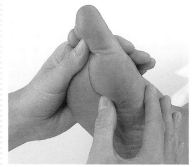

4 Work the air passages to stimulate them to clear themselves.

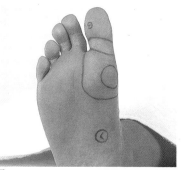

5 Work all the glands and take particular notice of any that seem especially tender.

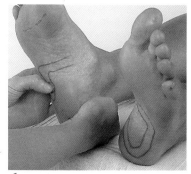

6 Work the ileo-caecal valve and the whole of the colon because this will help balance mucus levels and get rid of waste in the system.

RELIEVING HEADACHES AND NAUSEA

These two problems are often linked, with a blinding headache often contributing to feelings of nausea. Within the context of a full reflexology treatment, work for one or both as appropriate.

HEADACHES

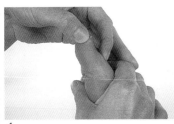

1 Work the hypothalamus reflex first, as this controls the release of endorphins for the relief of pain.

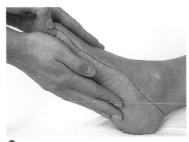

2 Work down the spine to take pressure away from the head. This will draw energy down the body and ground it.

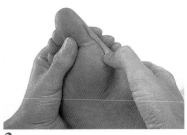

3 Work the cervical spine on the big toe. Work the neck of all the toes to relieve tension.

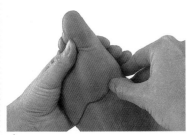

4 Work the diaphragm to encourage breathing.

NAUSEA

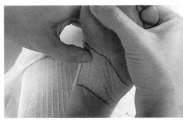

1 Work the whole abdomen, especially where it seems tender. Do this gently and with care.

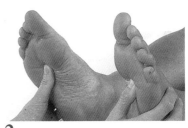

2 Do the solar plexus breathing exercise: take both feet together and position your thumbs in the centre of the diaphragm line. As your partner breathes in, press gently in with your thumbs, and, as they breathe out, release your thumbs. Repeat this several times following your partner's lead.

HELP WITH MENSTRUAL AND REPRODUCTIVE PROBLEMS

Work the whole reproductive system on the sides and top of the heel, as all parts work together.

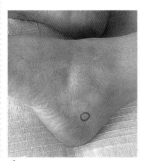

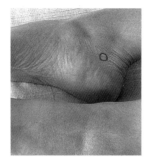

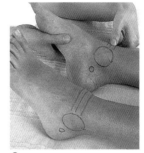

1 Work the ovaries or testes on the outside of the feet.

2 Work the uterus or prostate gland on the inside of the feet.

3 Work the fallopian tubes or vas deferens across the top of the ankle.

SELF-HELP: Refer to the hand chart at the back of the book to locate the ovaries or testes, and work this reflex on both hands. Then work the uterus or prostate gland, and finally the fallopian tubes or vas deferens.

MENSTRUAL CRAMPS

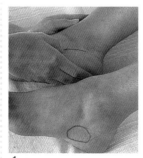

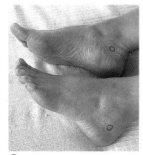

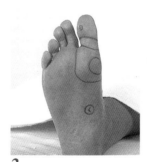

1 Work the lower spine for nerves to the uterus.

2 Work the uterus reflex on the inside of the feet.

3 Work the glands on both feet.

PAINFUL BREASTS

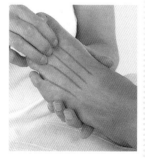

Fingerwalk up the chest area on top of the foot with three fingers together.

HELP WITH COLDS, SORE THROATS AND SINUS PROBLEMS

Colds, sore throats and sinus problems all affect the respiratory system. To stimulate them to clear themselves, you need to work all the toes and chest area.

COLDS

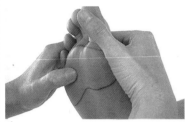

1 Work the chest to encourage clear breathing.

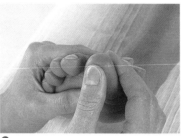

2 Beginning with the big toe, work the tops of all the toes to clear the sinuses. Then pinpoint the pituitary gland in the centre of the prints of both big toes to stimulate the endocrine system.

SORE THROATS

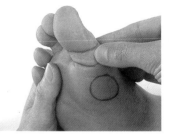

1 Work the upper lymph system, and then work the throat on the neck, and the thymus gland for the immune system.

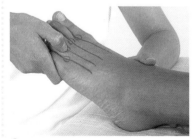

3 Work the upper lymph system to stimulate the immune system.

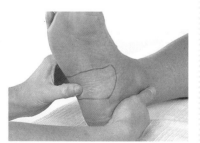

4 Work the small intestines to aid elimination of toxins and uptake of nutrients. Then work the colon to aid elimination.

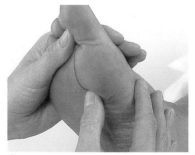

2 Work the trachea and the larynx to stimulate them to clear and heal.

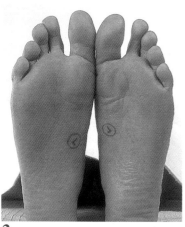

3 Rotate the adrenal reflex in the direction of the arrow.

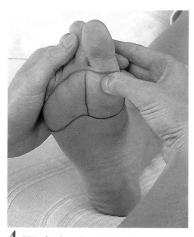

4 Work the thyroid helper area in the section of the chest under the big toe. Then work the whole chest area for the entire respiratory system.

SINUS PROBLEMS

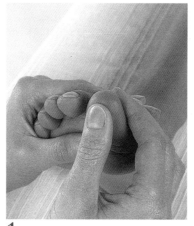

1 Work all the toes, especially the sinus reflexes to stimulate them to clear themselves.

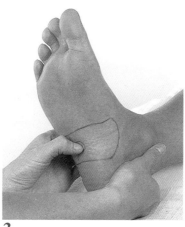

3 Pinpoint the ileo-caecal valve to balance mucus levels.

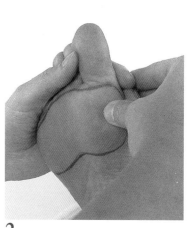

2 Work the whole chest area to aid respiration.

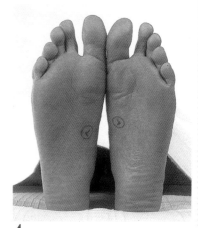

4 Rotate the adrenal reflex to reduce inflammation.

IMPROVING THE DIGESTION

The digestive system is a complex one with many and varied functions. It can be easily affected by stress and tension and, in the context of a full reflexology routine, particular attention can be given to the following areas.

INDIGESTION

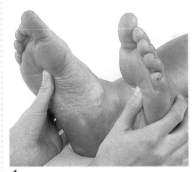

1 Work the solar plexus to relax the nerves to the stomach.

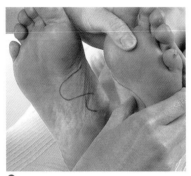

2 Work the stomach, where digestion really begins.

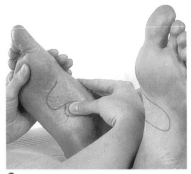

3 Then work the duodenum, the first section of the small intestines.

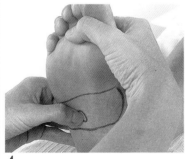

4 Work the liver and the gall bladder: the liver area is shown above, with the thumb rotating on the gall bladder reflex. These deal with digestion of fats.

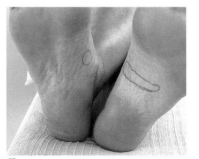

5 Work the pancreas which regulates blood sugar levels and aids digestion.

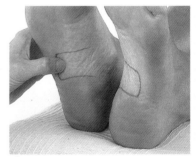

6 Work the small intestines where nutrients are absorbed. If there is bloatedness work the colon. (See the sequence for constipation opposite.)

CONSTIPATION

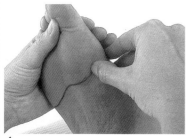

1 Work the diaphragm to relax the abdomen.

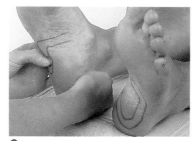

2 Pinpoint the ileo-caecal valve, which links small and large intestines.

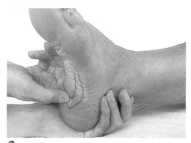

3 Work the colon or large intestine, especially the descending and sigmoid colon. This can become congested.

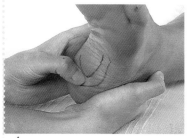

4 Pinpoint the sigmoid flexure. Being a bend, this can become congested.

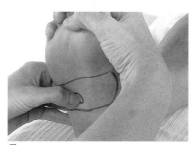

5 Work the liver and gall bladder: the liver area is shown above, with the thumb rotating on the gall bladder reflex.

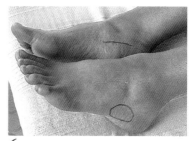

6 Work the lower spine and its helper areas for the nerve supply to the colon.

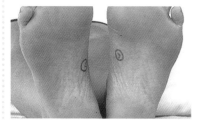

7 Work the adrenals for muscle tone. Rotate the reflex with your thumb in the direction of the arrows.

SELF-HELP:
Work the diaphragm to relax the abdomen and work the reflexes as described for the feet.

FOOT CHARTS

The foot charts are only guidelines for interpretation. When you find a tender or congested part of the foot you may look for that part on the charts and see approximately which reflex the tenderness lies on. This is only a rough guide because every pair of feet are different and will not be the same shape as your chart. Also, the charts are two-dimensional and your body is three-dimensional and therefore the reflexes on your feet reflect this. In reality your organs overlap each other, whereas the charts are much simplified for clarity, to give an idea of where things are.

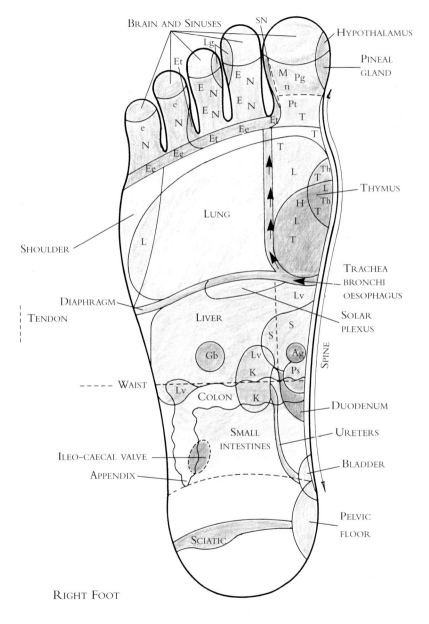

RIGHT FOOT

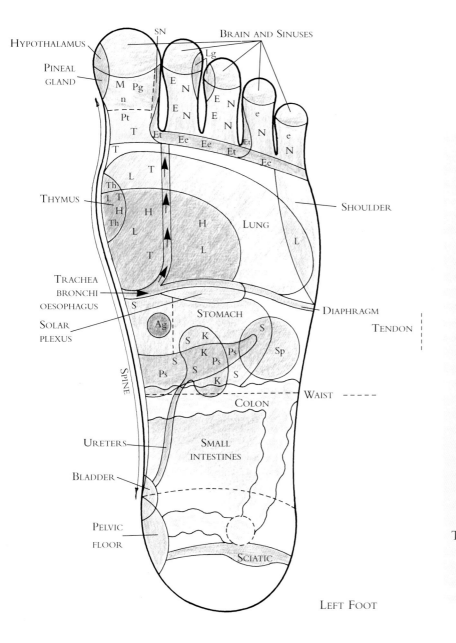

LEFT FOOT

KEY:

Ag Adrenal glands
e Ears
Et Eustachian tubes
Ee Eye/Ear helper
E Eyes
Gb Gall bladder
H Heart
K Kidneys
Lg Lachrymal glands
Lv Liver
L Lungs
M Mouth
N Neck
n Nose
Ps Pancreas
Pt Para-thyroid
Pg Pituitary glands
SN Side of neck
Sp Spleen
S Stomach
Tb Trachea bronchi oesophagus
th Thymus
T Thyroid

TOP AND SIDES OF FOOT

The spinal reflex (bottom) is especially important and should always be massaged, and the reflex worked thoroughly. Not only is our spinal column our main boney support but it also contains the spinal cord, and through the central nervous system the whole body may be treated on the spinal reflex.

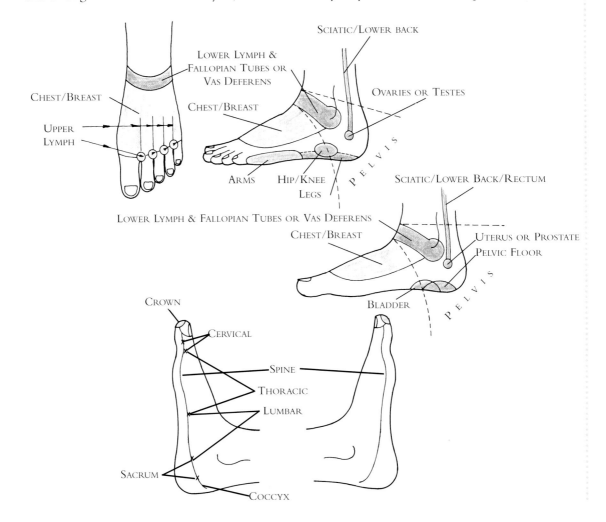

HAND CHARTS

The hands reflect all the body, as do the feet. They are a very different shape to feet, but once you have adjusted to that and learnt the basic layout, the location of reflexes is quite straightforward. Use the reflexes on the hand when you cannot work the feet for any reason. This may be the accessibility of hands rather than feet, or damage or disease to the feet, for example.

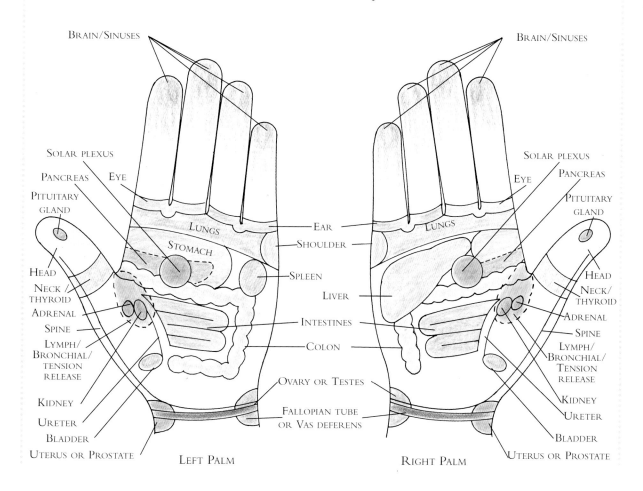

BRAIN/SINUSES

SOLAR PLEXUS
PANCREAS
EYE
PITUITARY GLAND
LUNGS
STOMACH
EAR
SHOULDER
HEAD
NECK / THYROID
SPLEEN
ADRENAL
SPINE
LYMPH/ BRONCHIAL/ TENSION RELEASE
LIVER
INTESTINES
COLON
KIDNEY
URETER
OVARY OR TESTES
BLADDER
FALLOPIAN TUBE OR VAS DEFERENS
UTERUS OR PROSTATE
LEFT PALM

BRAIN/SINUSES

SOLAR PLEXUS
PANCREAS
EYE
PITUITARY GLAND
LUNGS
HEAD
NECK/ THYROID
ADRENAL
SPINE
LYMPH/ BRONCHIAL/ TENSION RELEASE
KIDNEY
URETER
BLADDER
UTERUS OR PROSTATE
RIGHT PALM

Useful Addresses

MASSAGE

UK

The Massage Training Institute/
The Academy of On-site Massage
24 Brunswick Square
Hove
BN13 1EH

London College of Massage
5 Newman Passage
London
W1P 3PF

Clare Maxwell-Hudson Massage
Training Centre
PO Box 457
London
NW2 4BR

The School of Holistic Massage
c/o Nitya Lacroix
75 Dresden Road
London
N19 3BG

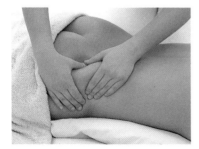

US

American Massage Therapy
Association
820 Davies Street, Suite 100
Evanston
IL 60201

Pacific School of Massage and
Healing Arts
44800 Fish Rock Road
Gualala
CA 95445

Body Therapy Center
368 California Avenue
Palo Alto.
CA 94306

AUSTRALIA

Association of Massage Therapists
3/33 Denham Street
Bondi
New South Wales

SHIATSU

UK

The British School of Shiatsu-Do
3rd Floor
130-132 Tooley Street
London
SE1 2TU

The Shiatsu Society
Interchange Studios
Dalby Street
London
NW5 3NQ

The European Shiatsu School
Central Administration
Highbanks
Lockeridge
Marlborough
Wiltshire
SN8 4EQ

US

International School of Shiatsu
10 South Clinton Street, Suite 300
Doylestown
PA 18901

School of Shiatsu and Massage at
Harbin Hot Springs
PO Box 889
Middletown
CA 95461

AUSTRALIA

The Shiatsu Therapy Association of
Australia
2 Caminoley Wynd
Templestowe
Victoria 3106

Australian Natural Therapies
Association Ltd.
Suite 1, 2nd Floor
468–472 George Street
(PO Box A964)
Sydney
New South Wales 2000

AROMATHERAPY

UK
International Society of Professional
Aromatherapists
The Hinckley and District Hospital
Mount Road
Hinckley
Leicestershire
LE10 1AG

International Federation of
Aromatherapists
4 Eastmearn Road
Dulwich
London
SE21 8HA

US
Institute of Aromatherapy
3108 Route 10
West Denville
NJ 07834

Aromatherapy School and Herbal
Studies
219 Carl Street
San Fransisco
CA 94117

AUSTRALIA
Australian School of Awareness
251 Dorset Road
Croydon
Victoria 3136

International Federation of
Aromatherapists
83 Riversdale Road
Hawthorn
Victoria 3122

REFLEXOLOGY

UK
Association of Reflexologists
27 Old Gloucester Street
London
W1N 3XX

Holistic Association of Reflexologists
92 Sheering Road
Old Harrow
Essex
CM17 0JW

The British Reflexology Association
12 Pond Road
London
SE3 6JL

US
International Institute of Reflexology
PO Box 12462
St Petersburg,
FL 33733

Reflexology Center
Scarborough Professional Center
136 Route One
Scarborough
ME 04074

AUSTRALIA
Reflexology Association of Australia
15 Kedumba Crescent
Turramurra
New South Wales 2074

RASA (Australia)
73 Illawong Way
Karand Downs
Brisbane
Queensland 4306

Australian School of Reflexology and
Relaxation
165 Progress Road
Eltham North
Victoria 3095

The publishers would like to thank
the following photographers for the
use of their pictures: Michelle Garrett,
Alistair Hughes, Lucy Mason and
Debbie Patterson.

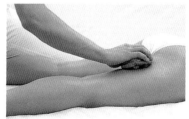

INDEX

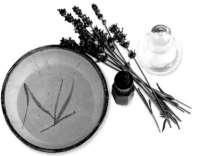

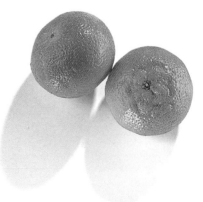

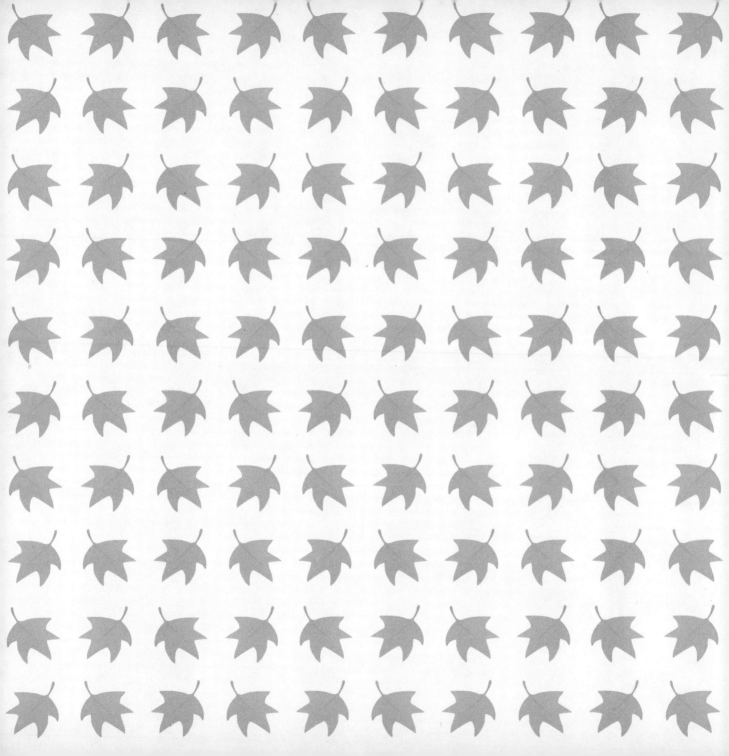